Sleep Well, Sleep Deep

Sleep Well, Sleep Deep

Alex Lukeman, Ph.D.

M. Evans and Company, Inc.
New York

M. Evans and Company, Inc.
216 East 49th Street
New York, New York 10017

Book design and typesetting by Rik Lain Schell

Printed in the United States of America

9 8 7 6 5 4 3 2 1

Many thanks to Noah and Gayle.

CONTENTS

INTRODUCTION

Can't sleep? You have plenty of company. Over fifty-three million people in our country don't get enough sleep. Over thirty million suffer from sleeping disorders like insomnia and sleepwalking. If you are tired of sleepless nights, you've come to the right place. *Sleep Well, Sleep Deep* shows how sleeping well can change your life. It contains up-to-date information on the latest research and thinking about sleep and sleep disorders. It presents simple, concrete steps to help you take your sleeping life into your own hands.

Sleep is one of those common threads in the tapestry of human experience that unites us all, like birth and death. Prophecy, scientific discoveries, strange and beautiful dreams, mystical experiences and murderous plots have all been associated with sleep. We are fascinated by sleep. We long for the bliss and renewal sleep can provide. We spend more than a third of our lives in it. Yet many of us are exhausted and ill prepared for our daily life, because restful sleep eludes us.

Sleep Well, Sleep Deep reveals the mysteries of sleep. It gives you practical advice about what to do when you can't sleep, what you should know about sleeping pills and other medications, what to do when your child can't sleep, and more. It talks about sleep problems and disorders and the mysterious world of dreams and dreaming. There is a chapter dedicated to practical self-hypnosis for stress relief and healthful sleep, useful for any-

1

one who has difficulty sleeping or is feeling stressed or pressured in life. Woven throughout the book are bits of myth and story that speak to us about sleep. Tips for dealing with common sleeping problems like jet lag or driver fatigue are included.

Sleep deprivation is a pervasive and destructive force. It is a hidden killer in our society, responsible for countless human tragedies only hinted at in brief filler segments seen on the evening news. Loss of sleep has devastating effects on our private lives and on the health of the nation's business and economy. Just as an example, over 100,000 car crashes a year can be directly attributed to drivers who haven't had enough sleep. We all know about the dangers of drunk drivers on our highways. How often do you hear about sleeping drivers? The National Highway Traffic Safety Administration estimates that as many as *one million* crashes a year may be due to fatigue. Did you know that there are very specific times of the day and night when you are much more likely to be at risk from someone falling asleep at the wheel? Did you know that *you* might be at risk of falling asleep at the wheel, without even being aware of the danger?

We can adopt an easy and powerful strategy for improving our health and the quality of our lives: we can learn how to sleep well. There's a lot of resistance in our culture to thinking about sleep as something desirable for its own sake. People who want to sleep are often seen as lazy and unreliable. "Sleeping on the job" is usually a sure recipe for getting fired. We are supposed to be alert, ready to take on any challenge of the workday at any time. We are often expected to work beyond "normal" hours, because the job demands it. Taking work home has become a way of life for many workers and managers. Jobs and financial survival depend on "going the extra mile," measured by our capacity to take on horrendous workloads and somehow meet ever more demanding deadlines.

In many corporations the relentless pursuit of productivity at all costs runs roughshod over any understanding or appreciation of the mental and physical stress that accompanies lost sleep. If the CEOs and corporate chairmen were truly aware of the costs their sleep-robbing policies create, they would change their tune. In the United States we are talking about an estimated $150 billion direct loss in productivity each year! Yes, that's billion with a *B*—direct losses resulting from bad workmanship, slow job performance, health care costs, accidents and bad PR for company products.

Many of us suffer needlessly from sleep deprivation. Many of us are not even aware of just how much lack of sleep is affecting us or that help is available for our problems. We don't know that we can make simple changes that lead to big results. We just assume that our particular circumstances don't allow for the kind of sleep we really desire.

We sense that the quality of our lives would be better if only we could get enough sleep, but many of us who don't sleep well have given up and learned to "live with it." I have good news for you if you are one of those people: you don't have to live with it. You can take charge of your sleep. There are specific steps and sleep strategies you can follow, resources you can call upon, experts to help you and a wealth of scientific research and traditional approaches to back you up. This book will show you what to do.

I wrote this for all of us who have had too many frustrating nights when we would have given almost anything for a good night's sleep. I hope it helps. May your sleep be peaceful and your dreams be sweet.

Alex Lukeman
Fort Collins, Colorado

CHAPTER ONE

SLEEPING WELL CAN CHANGE YOUR LIFE

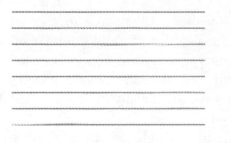

There is a dangerous, hidden problem in America that affects every one of us. It's not crime, pollution, or political scandal. It can be found in any home or family. It crosses all barriers of social status, ethnic background, economic resource, cultural preference, education and lifestyle. It affects young and old alike, opening the door to personal and social disaster. The problem is lack of sleep: more than a third of us don't get enough of it.

When we don't sleep well, bad things happen. The consequences of not getting enough sleep range from the annoying to the profound, from simple tiredness and irritability to grim accidents resulting in disfiguring injuries, disability, and death. In the workplace poor sleep causes escalating health costs, job losses, bitter arguments among co-workers, poor workmanship, low productivity, and bad management decisions. From a corporate standpoint it's a disaster; from a personal standpoint it's even worse.

Are you one of the millions who has trouble getting to sleep? One of millions more who goes to sleep with relative ease but wakes throughout the night and finally gives up at three or four in the morning? Are you tired during the day, falling asleep at work, struggling to keep awake? Do you spend frustrating nights restlessly tossing about on your crumpled sheets?

Sleep is the foundation of well-being, affecting every aspect of our lives. On any given night in America up to seventy million people have trouble sleeping. More women are affected with sleeplessness than men. We don't get enough sleep, and the quality of what sleep we do get is far from ideal.

Call me a dreamer: I believe it's possible to sleep well. Learning how to do it is one of the most effective ways available to us for improving our health and well-being. By taking charge of our sleep we take charge of a third of our lives. If we can make that third as restful and refreshing as possible, the other two-thirds—the part we are usually most concerned with—will naturally flourish as a result.

If you are one of the multitudes who don't sleep well there is something you can do about it. It won't cost you much except some of your time and attention to make things better. You simply need to discover what has to change so that your natural pattern of restful sleep can assert itself. That is why this book was written—to help you make the change.

At this very moment countless numbers of people are quietly asleep all over the world. For these lucky ones, sleep brings rest, relaxation, health, and relief from all the stressful trials of life. These peaceful sleepers are truly fortunate: everyone else trying to sleep is fitfully drifting in and out of consciousness and desperately wishing they could "just get a good night's sleep."

This entire book is about getting a good night's sleep. If you are someone who needs to get more sleep or has any kind of sleeping problem, then keep reading. The chances are you will find what you need to know to help improve your sleep somewhere along the way.

Sleep is much more than lying down and waking up. To discover what is causing your sleep problem and fix it, it helps to understand something about the nature of sleep as well as the kinds of things that disrupt it. Throughout the following pages you will find many different ideas and facts about sleep. You will also find practical and tested suggestions for identifying and fixing sleep problems of all types and descriptions. You are likely to find your particular situation described. If you have a specific problem in mind, like jet lag or sleepwalking, look in the index and you will be guided to areas and pages within the book that deal with your particular interest or concern.

WHAT IS SLEEP?

The language of sleep research can be confusing. You don't need to know it, but you do need to know something about how sleep works. You need to be familiar with the underlying mechanisms and physiology of sleep. You wouldn't expect a mechanic to repair your car without understanding the underlying principles of how it all works—the same is true for fixing sleep problems. Appreciating a few basic facts about sleep helps us devise strategies for improving it.

In this chapter I'm going to talk about sleep without getting too technical about it. I'm going to talk about our natural rhythms of sleep and wakefulness and why we should know about them. You'll find strategies and ideas in here about how to deal with problems caused by getting out of step with those rhythms. I promise not to get into too much detail, just enough to provide the kind of background information you need to help you build a successful strategy for better sleep.

Why do we need to sleep, and why can't we just find ways to do without it? What is this mysterious thing that literally takes up a full third of all our years? Why do we find ourselves confused, angry, and overwhelmed when we don't get the sleep we need? Without sleep we quickly lose the joy of life, our ability to work and play with ease and competence, our margin of safety in making critical judgments and decisions, even our sense of self as whole, productive, and balanced human beings.

In ancient Greece the god of sleep was named Hypnos. Hypnos was sometimes represented as carrying a bouquet of opium-laden poppy flowers. Opium was a very effective aid to sleep in olden times. Hypnos had a darker twin brother, Thanatos, who brought sleep of an eternal nature. It made sense to the Greeks to suppose that death and sleep were intimately related. They could see the sleeper's loss of outward consciousness and sensibility to the outer world and thought of it as a kind of temporary version of life's end. They couldn't know that the mind is far from unconscious during sleep. Our waking mind may not be aware of it, but sleep is far more than rest. It is a complex neural and physiological process that moves through predictable cycles of greater and lesser activity.

There has always been a lot of controversy among scientists and sleep researchers about the exact function of sleep. There are many theories and few facts. In most ways sleep is still the mystery it always was, in spite of years of research and study. From a scientific standpoint only a few things can be said with certainty about sleep.

All of us typically go through four stages of sleep in any given sleep cycle, and move through four or five cycles each night. Each cycle tends to last about ninety minutes or so. All of our senses are still functioning as we sleep, although at a greatly reduced level. Part of our brain remains awake and sends us signals of alarm if something goes wrong. Anyone who has awakened to the sound of a baby's cry or a strange sound in the night knows this is true. In the old days of saber-toothed tigers and other hungry predators, sleep was a dangerous thing. In our modern era there are still plenty of reasons to wake quickly if needed. Sleep still makes us vulnerable to danger. Even though we have come a long way from the cave dwellings of our primitive ancestors (although some might take issue with that), we still retain a built-in warning system that wakes us instantly at any sign of trouble or danger.

Some years ago I was living in New York City, on the Upper West Side in a ground-floor apartment. One night my wife and I were peacefully sleeping when I suddenly awoke. A rush of adrenaline surged through me, and I sat straight up in bed in the dark room. Standing at the foot of the bed was a large man, wearing a black ski mask and dressed completely in black, as if he had just stepped out of a bad Ninja movie. What a shock!

I'd love to say that I jumped out of bed and subdued the intruder with several well-placed Chuck Norris moves, but in reality I was momentarily stunned and immovable. By the time I realized this apparition was a burglar and that I ought to do something, he was gone, out the door and into the night. Later I couldn't help thinking I wouldn't have done very well in the saber-toothed tiger days.

The old built-in panic button brain mechanism still works, but it doesn't guarantee our survival. Sleep may suddenly vanish, but we are usually no longer well prepared for battle or flight when the alarms kick in. What we do once we wake up depends on more than just alertness. If we are sleep deprived, no amount of training or psychological preparation will save the day.

Whether we wake up or not depends on how the "sleeping" brain interprets the sounds around us. Even when deeply asleep, some part of the brain is listening. Recent research at Johns Hopkins University seems to indicate that there may be several different areas of the brain that monitor and evaluate sounds when we sleep, ignoring some, waking us gently for others, or throwing us into a state of adrenaline panic when danger appears. It's possible to defeat our internal warning system with drugs or alcohol, exhaustion or medication.

From a subjective, personal point of view, we all know what sleep is about. Just ask anyone who hasn't been able to sleep lately! We need to sleep to feel well, to rejuvenate our energy and rest our minds from the challenges and events of the day. Sleep maintains memory and helps the brain store, process, and integrate new information. Perhaps this is the real reason we have to sleep, but no one really knows.

Sleep is always associated with recovery from illness. It is a natural response to injury and trauma. While we sleep, the energy that would normally go toward waking functions becomes available for healing and rejuvenation. Sleep also acts to restore the clear function of our consciousness. If we are performing some highly task-oriented activity requiring very high mental attention, like tracking planes on a radar screen or focusing on very complex tasks with large information content, we need more sleep.

Researchers have explored and discovered the physiological mechanism of sleep up to a point, but it is still not yet fully understood. Modern sleep research focuses on complex hormonal secretion sequences, biochemical compounds and amino acids called neurotransmitters, as the biological key to sleep. Contemporary drug and herbal therapies zero in on these compounds and hormones as a means of promoting sleep. We'll look at these in detail later on, in chapter 5.

Sleep starts very early. In the womb the fetus is dreaming and sleeping most of the time, integrating neural circuits and preparing for entry into life. Did you know that the fetus sleeps and dreams? In infancy and early childhood, sleep is a critical piece of the learning and integration process our brains must experience for healthy and normal growth. This is one reason infants sleep so much at first. As we grow older the length of necessary daily sleep shortens. By age ten or so we are down to around ten hours of sleep a night for best functioning and health. By age twenty, we've moved closer to the eight hours that is the norm for most. That remains the usual pattern until we reach middle age. Sometime around fifty, we begin to sleep less, and the quality of our sleep may begin to change. When we reach our elder years, we may not sleep well at all and much less than we used to. Fortunately there are things we can do about this: we'll look at many sleep problems and "fixes" later on in the book, including getting older and maintaining sleep.

Where can we discover what is happening in our bodies and minds during sleep? If you lived in ancient Greece, you could seek advice from the oracle at Delphi. At Delphi and in other ritually consecrated and sacred temples, the sleeper attempted to commune with the gods, usually through a dream.

The modern equivalent of Delphi is found in our current temples of sleep, called "sleep labs." In sleep labs subjects are carefully observed while sleeping, just as you would expect. They are hooked up to an array of sophisticated equipment that measures a multitude of physical and neurological functions. The primary instrument used in this kind of sleep research is the EEG, or electroencephalogram machine, which records minute electrical variations produced in the brain during different stages of sleep. These appear on a paper printout as a series of inked lines or are transmitted directly to a computer for recording and analysis. Other similar machines measure temperature and respiratory changes, physical movements, and more. The wealth of data produced by the machines reveals a moderately clear picture of what is happening when we sleep, at least as far as giving us an electrical map of brain and physical activity, and a set of measurements of the process.

ALL YOU REALLY NEED TO KNOW ABOUT BRAIN WAVES AND SLEEP

The EEG reveals four distinct "wave" patterns of activity in the brain. If you were hooked up right now to an EEG it would show a very characteristic pattern, instantly telling the trained researcher that you are awake (at least I hope you are still awake after reading this far!). The researcher would not need to be in the same room with you or even need to directly observe you. The EEG would make the state of your waking consciousness very clear. It would also show a distinct pattern indicating the movement of your eyes as they scan back and forth across this page as you are reading. This charting of eye movements becomes significant at a later stage of sleep.

The pattern of electrical waves in the brain when we are awake is called *beta*. Beta waves are rapid in nature. When we lie down to sleep, beta waves begin to slow to alpha waves. These are the first signs of sleep, marking a transitional zone to deeper levels. When alpha waves appear on the EEG we are not asleep, but are calm and relaxed. Alpha waves are sought after in biofeedback and meditative techniques you may have heard about. Many stress-relief programs seek to induce an alpha state of consciousness. Alpha waves are slower in frequency than beta and show a characteristic pattern produced by a higher-voltage reading than beta.

True sleep begins with the appearance on the EEG of theta waves. Theta waves mark Stage 1 sleep (light sleep). With the appearance of other characteristic electrical variations in the EEG patterns, called "sleep spindles," we slip into Stage 2. Ten or fifteen minutes later the brain waves change again and delta patterns appear, mixed with theta. Delta waves are slower than the others, of longer duration. This is Stage 3. Finally the theta waves disappear entirely and only the slow, delta waves remain. This is Stage 4, deep sleep. Stage 4 sleep is also known as slow-wave sleep. There are four or five full cycles of this repetitive cycling through the brain-wave patterns, going in and going out of deep sleep, throughout the night.

About an hour and a half after we fall asleep, a new pattern appears. This is called REM sleep, and it is the time of dreams. REM stands for "Rapid Eye Movement," because we can observe the eyes of the sleeper moving and tracking during this phase of sleep. This can also be seen in animals. Have you ever watched your cat or dog when they are asleep? Every dog owner has thought that Old Spot was probably chasing rabbits in some field of dreams, and Tabby is most likely after that pesky mouse. Understanding the cycle of brain waves gives us a kind of electrical map of brain activity during sleep. The map shows the brain is far from idle while sleeping.

THE BIOLOGICAL SLEEP CLOCK

With practice we can learn to enter states of deep relaxation that allow us to alter our brain-wave activity; we can use that kind of technique to trigger sleep. It is possible to modify brain-wave patterns while awake, especially shifting from beta to alpha patterns. There are some individuals, practiced in forms of meditation, who are able to maintain conscious awareness even in theta and delta states. Usually people who can do this apparently impossible feat are skilled in disciplined spiritual meditation practices. They have learned to consciously enter a state of brain-wave activity that for most of us would mean we were sound asleep. These folks are definitely the exception to the rule. A self-relaxation exercise is given later in the book, in chapter 7, that can help you enter an alpha state.

There's more to sleep and sleeping well than brain waves. There is another key component of sleep physiology that is often behind many of our sleeping problems. It can have immediate effects on the way we feel and on the quality of our lives: it's our internal biological clock. Our clock tells us when it's time to sleep and when it's time to get up. It's this clock that gets confused when we go on night shifts or fly to Hawaii, or when we accidentally reprogram ourselves to stay up late. If the clock says it's time to sleep, we'd better pay attention or there will be consequences. The clock is something we can work with and even modify.

There are three different kinds of animals in the world, and humans are almost one of them. There are animals that normally awaken and function in the dark, there are animals that only come out during the day, and there are animals that come out at dawn and at dusk. Humans have developed the ability to do any of these things, but we are primarily daytime creatures. Our internal clocks are geared to the hours of sunlight and are triggered and reset by variations of light and dark. Biological cycles cued by darkness and light, called circadian rhythms, rule our lives. *Circadian* is formed from the Latin words *circa* (about) and *dies* (day). In other words, our natural cycle of internal biological rhythms is "about a day." When these rhythms are functioning without interference, we are in an easy and natural cycle of wakefulness and sleep, rest and activity, tiredness and alertness. When the rhythms are disturbed, as happens all too easily in our modern society, things go awry and we are suddenly dealing with fatigue, sleeplessness, and reduced mental abilities. Circadian rhythms regulate all the major functions of our body, including the production of hormones and steroids, the onset and completion of sleep, body temperature, heart rate, the production of urine, and more. Each function has its own distinct rhythm, its own cycle and timing.

It's easy for the rhythms to get pushed too far from normal. In a world of high-speed air travel, overtime, night shifts, and "cost effective" shift rotations, one of the first things to go is our natural sense of timing for sleep and wakefulness. When this is coupled with work that requires critical decision making and attention to detail, rigid deadlines, extended working hours, and pressure to "get the job done," the result is often disaster. When circadian rhythms are disrupted, the result is internal confusion. This often leads to sleep deprivation.

SLEEP DEPRIVATION

Many terrible disasters can be laid directly at the feet of sleep loss and disrupted circadian "clocks." When the nuclear reactor at Chernobyl exploded, it poisoned thousands of square miles with radioactive fallout, sent a cloud of radioactivity over Europe and around the world, and set in motion a chain of events leading to economic disaster, hardship, and disease that continues to this day. The workers at Chernobyl had been on duty for eighteen hours or more. They were supposed to be performing a routine series of safety checks, shutting down certain systems and activating others. The operating procedures were clear and took into account the need to activate backup and safety systems while the maintenance work was being carried out. The workers did exactly the wrong thing, shutting down critical systems in the belief that they were doing the opposite. That is very typical of what happens when we are deprived of sleep. We make decisions that seem perfectly clear and correct, but which are in reality terribly wrong.

Another example of what happens when people don't get enough sleep is the explosion of the *Challenger* space shuttle. This tragic event could easily have been prevented. Engineers and supervisors had been up for as much as fifty hours straight prior to the launch and were under enormous pressure from Washington and top levels of NASA to keep to the schedule. Their decisions were flawed by their inability to think clearly, a direct result of their collective lack of sleep. Warnings from junior engineers that there could be a serious problem were ignored. All of the information regarding the conditions that actually caused the explosion was available to the decision makers, but was glossed over or dismissed. If these people had not been sleep deprived, it is probable that the explosion would not have taken place. Someone would have paid attention to the danger and aborted the launch.

Sleep deprivation makes it impossible to think clearly, even though our subjective feeling may be that everything is fine! We say to ourselves, "I'm just a little tired," but our attention becomes narrowed and focused in ways that are extremely limiting and often dangerous to our safety and well-being. Information that is perfectly clear to the rested mind becomes unseen, unheard, and unavailable. So, if you find yourself waiting behind someone who's not moving at the green light, don't get impatient: they're probably asleep. Next time it might be you!

Lack of sleep can be used as a tactic to manipulate outcomes in negotiations. It's not by accident that labor mediators often achieve agreements in the wee hours of the morning, after days of prolonged and detailed meetings. It's standard practice to get participants so tired that difficult details become lost in the haze of sleeplessness and fatigue.

Sleep deprivation is one of a selection of standard psychological tactics sometimes employed by police in armed confrontations. It doesn't always work, and I personally think it is usually a serious mistake, because it can easily backfire. The thinking behind it is geared toward distracting, confusing, and wearing down the target of government or police attention. You may recall the events at Waco, Texas, when the confrontation with the Branch Davidian cult came to a fiery end. I wonder if a peaceful resolution might have been achieved if the government had refrained from making normal sleep impossible for the people within the compound? Tactics included endless playing of abrasive and loud music and sounds throughout the night, every night, for weeks on end. When people can't think straight because of sleep deprivation, they make bad decisions. They most certainly do not make reasonable ones.

When the mind is deprived of sleep long enough, it will sleep regardless of imminent physical danger or the need to stay alert for survival. There are many stories told by combat veterans of falling asleep even though their lives and the lives of their buddies depended on staying awake. Here's a brief Vietnam story from an ex–combat Marine named Eddie that illustrates this truth:

> We were on patrol all day and up fifty percent of every night. Everyone tended to fall asleep on post. . . . We were in two-man foxholes. I was with a new guy. It was my watch and I was dozing off, and the new guy—he was from Texas, the new guy in my outfit. It was my watch and I dozed off—and when I woke up I was looking at the business end of an M-14. He said, "Don't you ever f---ing do that again." I never did!

Eddie was lucky it was just the "new guy" who was pointing a rifle at him. It could just as easily have been someone who wanted to kill him. Even the reality of constant danger and possible death couldn't keep an experienced combat soldier like Eddie awake.

Sleep will overwhelm us if we have pushed the envelope too far, and we cannot do a thing about it. A study done in Germany not too long ago is particularly revealing. A subject was kept awake until well past the threshold of sleep deprivation, wired up to a portable EEG, placed in a high-speed car, and sent off down the Autobahn to determine how he would respond while driving under the effects of lost sleep. According to the information recorded by the researchers, the driver was actually asleep at the wheel for as long as twenty minutes at a time! During this time he continued to negotiate turns, maintain control of the car, and motor on down the road!

The name for this phenomenon is Automatic Behavior Syndrome. It occurs when we are seriously sleep deprived. A person affected with ABS continues to look as if they are awake and performing the routine action, whatever it is. It could be driving to work. It could be operating a piece of machinery or jockeying a big semi down the highway. The person's eyes are open, but no one is home! As soon as something a little out of the ordinary occurs, trouble happens. The truck driver doesn't see a turn and hurtles off the road. The locomotive engineer doesn't see a red signal and plows into the rear of a passenger train. The anesthesiologist fails to see that a patient's oxygen level is dangerously depleted and brain death results.

A very dangerous effect of sleep deprivation is something called "microsleep." Microsleep doesn't last as long as Automatic Behavior Syndrome, but it's similar in its potential for lethal results. When we are sleep deprived beyond the brain's tolerance, we will go into microsleep, and we cannot avoid it. Microsleep means that the brain actually sleeps for very brief periods of time. For fifteen or twenty seconds, perhaps longer, we will not respond to the normal stimuli of our environment.

I don't know about you, but I find this a little unsettling. If you think about it, a car going seventy-five miles per hour (the current speed limit on the interstate in my home state of Colorado) will travel one hundred ten feet in one second. If the car is in good mechanical condition and on a level, smooth surface with no other factors (like wind or rain) present, then it's reasonable to assume it can travel four to five hundred feet in a straight line with no input from the driver. After that, various factors begin to divert the car from its straight course: it will begin to drift to the side, ever so slightly. At seventy-five miles per hour mph it will begin to drift after four or five seconds, perhaps. If not corrected, in another five seconds it will have traveled another five hundred fifty feet and, chances are, will be heading off the road. In fifteen seconds the vehicle will have traveled considerably more than the length of five football fields and will be well off the road or close to it.

If you are behind the wheel of a car going seventy-five and you slip into a microsleep of fifteen or twenty seconds, chances are good you will not wake up again.

Here's a brief list of things you can do to make sure you don't fall asleep at the wheel.

Staying Awake and Alive

—— Make sure you are rested and caught up on your sleep before you begin any long drive.

—— Take breaks: I like to take a break about every two or two and a half hours or so. Get out of the car. Move around, stretch, take a few deep breaths—you'll be more alert and ready for the next leg of the journey.

—— Learn to recognize the signs of a fatigue that is becoming dangerous. Frequent yawns, tired and itchy eyes, squirming around in your seat trying to get comfortable, finding yourself braking a little too hard, a little too late—if these things are happening, maybe you should start looking for that motel.

—— Don't trust the old tricks of opening the window or cranking up the radio to keep you awake. Yes, I've done it and so have you, but it doesn't really solve the problem. You are still very tired, and the fresh air won't keep you awake if microsleep hits you. If you are that tired, you need to quit for the day or at least pull over and take a nap—forty-five minutes is probably about right, not longer.

—— Plan your trip to include an overnight break if driving time is much more than nine or ten hours to your destination. Don't pull an all-day, all-nighter to get where you're going. That's a good way to increase the odds you will never arrive.

—— Don't rely on coffee or caffeine to keep you awake. You burn up your reserves and open the door to micro-sleep as you become progressively more tired. Same thing for having that pie and ice cream break to "keep going."

—— Try to avoid driving during the circadian low cycles, at around three o'clock in the morning or in the after-noon. There is a natural circadian "dip" that takes place at these times, when your body rhythms are at their lowest ebb of energy and alertness. When a dip is occurring you may be vulnerable to episodes of microsleep and errors of judgment, especially if you were a little tired when you started.

—— Don't even think about alcohol, cold medications, anti-histamines, or other drugs.

I remember once falling asleep at the wheel at about three in the morning and waking up as the car left the edge of the road. I was lucky, because I had just enough time to pull back onto the pavement. I was going over sixty-five and headed into thick woods. I was sixteen years old at the time, but I have never for-gotten that jolt as I realized I was about to crash into the trees! Youthful reaction time and luck saved me then, but what if it happened now? What if you fall asleep at the wheel? How's *your* reaction time these days?

Have I got your attention yet? Losing sleep can mean a lot more than irritability and poor job performance: it can mean your life. But, you say, I don't drive. This doesn't affect me.

That's not really true, because we live in a world where cars are an ever-present fact of life. I'd be very surprised if you never ride in a car, even if you are not driving. And what about airplanes, buses, boats, and trains? All of these vehicles have "drivers." The Exxon *Valdez* ran aground because the man steering the ship was asleep.

If nuclear reactors exploding, spaceships going down in flames, terrible carnage on the highway, and environmental disaster aren't enough to convince you that sleep deprivation can lead to very severe results, let me offer one more chilling possibility to think about. How much sleep has your surgeon, anesthesiologist, or emergency room staff been getting lately?

You have probably seen or read something about the problems caused by sleep deprivation for doctors who are going through their internships or residencies. The system of medical training and residency includes years of long and arduous shifts, frequently averaging eighty hours a week. These are the folks who tend to find themselves on the 3:00 A.M. shift in the ER. The hard truth is that doctors who are consistently deprived of adequate and regular sleep will make mistakes. Let's hope you and I will never need to be treated by someone who is at the end of a busy and demanding thirty or forty hours without more than a few stolen catnaps of ten or fifteen minutes.

There is a small bright spot here. Even when we are somewhat sleep deprived, there are periods when we are more alert and able to function well. Our circadian rhythms have highs and lows during the day, and we can take advantage of that fact when we are planning for something like surgery that requires skilled alertness. I strongly recommend that you schedule a key event like surgery for about 8:30 to 9:00 A.M. During this period the internal rhythms are at their peak, and they peak again at about the same time at night. The worst time is around three in the afternoon or early morning. Many people die in hospitals around these times because the life energies seem to be at their ebb during this period. It is a function of the circadian cycle.

Whether it's surgery or a flight to the coast, sitting at a blackjack table in Vegas, driving to work or simply wanting to be at your best, pay attention to this timing. Some people will naturally be a little later in hitting their peak, because their cycle is geared an hour or two later than the others, but the same principles apply. Avoid the down times of two to four in the afternoon and morning, and take advantage of the peak circadian energy to get things done.

SLEEP DEBT

In our society the norm is sleep deprivation, not regular and sufficient sleep. Almost all of us are operating with considerable "sleep debt." Sleep debt is a term coined by Dr. William Dement. Dr. Dement is director of the Sleep Disorders Clinic at Stanford University and heads the National Sleep Foundation, an excellent source of information about anything to do with sleep. When researchers say "sleep debt" they are talking about the accumulated effect of lost sleep. Sleep debt results from not having enough sleep over a period of time. Just like the balance on your credit card, you can "max out" and run out of resources. Sleep debt leads to gradually deteriorating mental and physical functions and an ever-increasing demand by the brain for sleep. To make things worse, we are almost always unable to really understand just how tired we are.

Sleep debt is sneaky and insidious. We may think we're fine, but as soon as the stimulation levels in our environment drop, we nod off very quickly. A monotonous speaker, a boring business meeting, a mediocre movie, a clichéd TV show (most of them, perhaps), a dull, uninteresting highway unrolling before you—all of these things and more can trigger a burst of sleep. There is almost nothing you can do about it if the debt is large enough.

Do you like to have an occasional glass of wine or a beer and then drive home? You may be able to easily handle one or two drinks without noticeable impairment of your abilities to think

21

and act. But if you are carrying a bit of sleep debt that one drink may hit you very hard and very quickly, and before you know it you're facing a DUI charge. It's not the alcohol so much as it is the sleep debt—your body simply can't handle the effect of the booze in the same way it can when you are rested and alert.

It's easy to tell if you are carrying sleep debt, now that you are aware of the possibility. There's a clear warning from your body. You're sitting at your desk, for example, when suddenly you are almost literally overwhelmed by a sense of drowsiness. You feel as if you really want to lie down. You have an uncontrollable urge to yawn deeply. That's a sign of sleep debt, even if it's nearing your regular bedtime. If it happens during the day, especially if it happens more than once, you're absolutely not getting enough sleep.

SHORT AND LONG SLEEPERS

Not too many years ago a flurry of scientific studies and theories suggested that we could all do with quite a bit less sleep than we were used to, as little as five to five and a half hours per day. This was touted as a wonderful breakthrough in the quality of life, because we would then have so much more time to do other things, like working or studying or watching movies or having sex. If we saved two and a half hours a day of sleep, this would add up to 17½ hours a week, 910 hours a year, or 63,700 hours over a seventy-year life span. Scientists love to throw numbers like this around. Who could argue with the idea of more available time to do things?

Alas, for almost everyone, the theories turn out to be impractical at best and destructive at worst, if actually put into practice. We can force ourselves to sleep less, reducing our sleeping time gradually until we reach the desired target of five and a half hours. But except for a group of people called "short sleepers" who already can do this naturally, the rest of us suffer serious effects. Our judgment deteriorates and we become irritable and angry. We make mistake after mistake: sex and any other kind of relationship activity becomes a memory (if we could remember, which we can't), and our lives contract as the brain shuts down more and more of the "unnecessary" attention to detail that fills our usual daily round.

We are naturally either short sleepers or long sleepers. Short sleepers are fine with five and a half hours of sleep. They do not understand why everyone isn't like them and really suspect that people who sleep longer are "just lazy." This can be a big problem if your boss or supervisor is a short sleeper, because he or she is liable to assume you can do just fine with five hours of sleep also and therefore have plenty of time to get that huge workload done. By far the majority of us are long sleepers, meaning we really must have seven and a half hours to nine and a half hours hours of sleep on a regular basis. If we don't get the sleep we need, we start to "lose it."

LARKS AND OWLS

Another interesting difference between us has to do with when we actually function best during the day. Some of us awaken early and do our best work in the morning; some sleep later and really don't come up to speed until later in the day. Sleep researchers call these two types "larks" and "owls." I don't know who coined the descriptions, but they generally fit: most of us are one or the other, though some fall in between.

If you are a "lark" (like me) you really feel best in the morning. That's the time to get your really serious and creative work out of the way, leaving the more mundane or routine stuff until later. Your day will probably end around ten or ten-thirty at night. If you are an "owl," like my wife, you want to sleep later in the morning. You don't really start to click until 11:00 A.M. or noon, and your best time to work is through the afternoon and into the early evening. You will stay up later—it's just not possible for you to go to sleep much before 11:00 P.M.

Sleep Well, Sleep Deep

Needless to say, this requires a bit of adaptation in relationship. I wonder how many marriages have come to grief because of mixing lark and owl? Which one are you? Here are a few simple questions you can ask yourself to find out.

A Brief Bird-Watcher's Guide

—— Do you like to get up before 7:00 A.M. in the morning and feel uncomfortable if you oversleep?

—— Does your best work get done in the morning or later in the day?

—— Do you feel as if you didn't get enough sleep if you get up much before 9:00 A.M.?

—— Do you usually go to bed by 10:30 or so, or do you usually stay up later?

—— Have you often felt out of step with people because you like to sleep late?

—— If you get up early, do you feel a little bit off all through the day?

Some people are not quite lark or owl and if you are one of these you will not have a strong opinion on these questions. Many of us tend to fall at the extremes. Larks are up early, so if you said "yes" to question one, you are definitely in the lark category. Larks do not feel good about sleeping late.

Question number two is a good indicator of your avian inclination. Larks are best in the morning: they are inspired then, have more energy and generally prefer to tackle the tough jobs right away. Owls, on the other hand, will put off working on anything serious until later in the day. After eleven or twelve they start to come on strong, and that will continue for most of the

24

afternoon. Take a look at your work habits, and you will have a good idea of which bird you are.

If you answered "yes" to number three, you are most likely an owl. Of course you may have a work schedule or some other factor that affects your answers (and when you have to get up or prefer to get up), but if you are on a normal day schedule this is a pretty good indicator of owlhood.

Number four is another strong indicator. Larks are pretty much done with the day at ten or ten-thirty. Owls keep going. As with all the other questions, this is just an indicator. But chances are if you are drawn to work like running a nightclub disco or tracking the movements of the stars, you are probably owl-inclined.

Questions five and six are both owl indicators, if you answered "yes." Owls don't quite fit in comfortably because everyone else seems to be getting up early and praising the virtues of the morning. The classic lark comment, designed to make you feel paranoid and guilty if it doesn't suit your temperament, is Benjamin Franklin's famous homily: "Early to bed and early to rise, makes a man healthy, wealthy, and wise." Remember that one? Old Ben had an attitude that makes owls feel sullen—after all, an owl doesn't feel at his or her best when rising early.

Whichever you are, honor it and don't try to change it around because of someone else's idea about when you should get up or go to bed. You may not have a lot of choice if you are working a regular job with regular hours, but if you can, let the natural order of things prevail. You probably have learned to adjust your sleep to your work schedule, but if and when that changes, the underlying pattern will emerge. Neither lark nor owl is a better way to be—it's just the way we are.

CIRCADIAN DISRUPTION

The frenetic, driven pace of modern business and the corporate workplace does not favor a regular schedule of eight hours of sleep. Perhaps the real villain is Thomas Edison, whose invention of the electric light forever changed the way business is done. Edison was a short sleeper, by all accounts, and claimed to sleep even less than he actually did. Some reports paint a picture of Edison as a somewhat opinionated workaholic who took a lot of short naps. Whatever the truth of Edison's sleeping patterns or his nature, the lightbulb banished the ancient rhythm of daylight and night and the presence of the sun in the sky as the prime factors in determining working hours and working rhythms.

Remember the biological clock? The key to setting or resetting the clock is light. The natural rhythm of our internal clock is "about a day"; actually, it's closer to twenty-five hours than twenty-four, but close enough. In controlled experiments in which subjects lived in environments completely isolated from the outer world cues we use to mark day and night, the internal clock gradually moved forward to about a twenty-five-hour-a-day period. In other words, our natural inclination is in a "clockwise" direction, forward, not back. This raises some practical questions for the workplace and the quality of our lives.

For example, suppose you are placed on a rotating shift that rotates counterclockwise? In other words, you start off on the night shift and then, after the prescribed period (days to weeks, depending on the company and location), you are rotated to an afternoon shift. This is followed by a morning shift and then, finally, by a night shift as the cycle starts to repeat. This kind of rotation goes against the clock, and is much harder to adjust to than an opposite pattern. For some reason the introduction of night shifts (a direct result of Edison's invention) and rotating shifts around the clock has traditionally been in a counterclockwise rotation. Trying to break this pattern in corporate America is like trying to walk to the moon. It is seemingly impossible to get management to understand that it is to their advantage to change direction and let their employees have an easier time of adjustment to the unnatural rhythms of nighttime production. If you work on a rotating shift that moves forward, you are the exception: count yourself lucky.

If you are one of the many who is forced to endure the constant reshuffling of your sleep patterns because of a rotating shift, you have my sympathy. You need more than sympathy to get the sleep you need. What can you do?

The best advice I can give you is mostly contained in chapter 2. Since you will often find yourself trying to sleep during the day or at times when others are wide awake and going about their daily routines, your sleeping environment is critical. Whatever it takes to make your bedroom dark and quiet, go for it. Make your hours as regular as possible. If you are a family person, then try to work in family time in some way that doesn't always take away from your sleeping time. Perhaps the best advice is this: get a different job. Easier said than done, but in the end it's the only way to really get settled into the kind of regular sleep pattern that supports your health and peace of mind.

JET LAG

When we're looking at how modern life shakes up the normal rhythms of things, maybe we should point our finger at the Wright brothers as well. Air travel is one of the worst culprits when it comes to causing lost sleep. If you have ever taken a long flight, especially across more than two or three time zones, you know what I mean. We even have that wonderfully descriptive term "jet lag" to describe the feeling.

Jet lag is what happens when your clock gets quickly and dramatically tossed into a different time zone. Your body feels as though it is lagging behind itself. Just as with the rotating shifts, going against the movement of the sun is harder. From Denver to Athens, heading east, is much more difficult than the return trip, when you are following the sun. The hard fact is that a long flight in either direction will act to disrupt the internal clock and set you up for unpleasant effects.

The problem, of course, is that when you arrive at your destination, your body clock is still ticking away just as it was some several hours earlier. It still thinks you are in your home area and expects to follow the same patterns of sleeping and waking, eating and working and resting. But wait—the sun is in the wrong place! It's night or it's high noon, but it should be something else, according to your inner rhythms.

Sensitivity to amounts of light is one of the triggering mechanisms of sleep. The exact place in the brain where this light sensitivity is registered might make a great answer to a trivia question or a question in a *Jeopardy* game or a crossword puzzle. It's called the suprachiasmatic nucleus, which loosely translates as "that bunch of cells over the X." The "X" in this case is the place where the optic nerves cross as they head on into the brain. The cluster of cells found in the suprachiasmatic nucleus registers minute changes of light transmitted from the eyes. These signals trigger the pineal gland, which in turn triggers chemical cascades of hormones, enzymes and amino acids to either wake you up or put you to sleep.

There's an interesting implication here, because if light is the trigger for sleep/wake changes, then perhaps we could use light to modify our sleep patterns in a conscious way and reset our biological clocks to prepare for the disruption of either night shifts or jet lag. In fact, we can do exactly that. It does take a clear program and intention to do it, but if we know that change is coming, we can make it a little easier on ourselves.

DEFEATING JET LAG

The idea of a biological clock that responds to cycles of light and dark dates back to 1728, when a French scientist named Jean de Marain took a mimosa plant and locked it up in a dark closet. The mimosa is noted for having leaves that open during the day and close at night. It was thought that the leaves simply were responding mechanically to the presence or absence of daylight. De Marain discovered that the leaves of his tormented plant continued to open and close in a daily rhythm that matched the ebb and flow of daylight, even when kept in complete darkness. History does not record whether or not the mimosa survived the experiment.

The human clock is likewise set to the particular rhythm of light and darkness found in our local environment. When we step off the plane in an environment that is hours ahead or behind in our usual relationship to the sun, the clock gets very confused. The circadian rhythm has been disrupted.

Changes from light to dark trigger the secretion of a hormone called melatonin from the pineal gland. You may have heard about melatonin. Health stores and even grocery stores now sell melatonin as a sleep aid. The secretion of melatonin, associated with the onset of darkness, appears to trigger a biochemical sequence that encourages sleep. Sleep patterns can be adjusted by suppressing the production of melatonin or increasing it. This can be handy if you have to attend an important business meeting in Singapore after a long flight, when your body thinks it ought to be asleep.

The key to naturally altering the sleep cycle initiated by the secretion of melatonin is light—lots of it. Melatonin secretion is suppressed if you are exposed to bright light, but it has to be very bright. Brightness is measured in a unit called the "lux." Normal daylight produces a reading of about 100,000 lux, but you don't need that much to affect melatonin. About 4,000 lux will do it. More is better. Of course, if you run down to your local light shop and ask for something that produces several thousand lux, they are liable to look at you very oddly and start inching toward the phone, just in case. Fortunately, some firms are beginning to produce something called a "light box" that can do the job.

The idea is to use bright light to reset your internal clock. If you expose yourself to bright light in the early evening, you delay the onset of sleep slightly. The later you do it, the more the delay. This requires some attention, however, because you could take it too far and begin to reverse the effect and start advancing the sleep time instead of retarding it.

Sleep Well, Sleep Deep

You probably don't want to be lugging around a big box full of fluorescent light bulbs on your business trip or vacation, so you need to prepare for the time shift before you leave. Ideally, you could gradually reset your internal clock to the correct local time at your destination, stepping off the plane fully synchronized to local rhythms and cycles of work, eating, rest, sleep, and wakefulness. By exposing yourself for fifteen or twenty minutes a day to very intense light for a period of several days before you depart, you can advance or retard the onset of the sleep cycle.

A simpler strategy, and perhaps the best, does not require a light box but does require attention and a desire to get the adjustment made before you go. This can be particularly useful for longer journeys and times when you know you will be spending a few days or more at your destination. Let's say you are going from San Francisco to Tokyo, where it is five hours earlier than in California. (We are talking about the position of the sun in relationship to your personal day, not the International Date Line, which would actually make it nineteen hours later.) You begin your preparation three days before. On the first day, stay up for two or three hours longer than normal. If your normal bedtime is 10 P.M., stay up until twelve or one in the morning. On the second day (the day before your flight), go to bed two hours earlier than normal, *i.e.*, at 8 P.M. The third day, in Tokyo, go to bed at your normal time. Presto! You're adjusted, or at least mostly so. You don't need to adjust your day exactly to the destination time, only within a couple of hours or so. That's good enough to avoid most of the effects of jet lag.

What if you are going the other way, for example, from San Francisco to London? There is an eight-hour difference between the two cities. Your normal 10 P.M. bedtime in San Francisco is 6 A.M. in London. That's not going to work very well, especially if you arrive in the morning when your body thinks you should be sound asleep. You must back up your bedtime, which takes a little doing. I recommend spending more time to adjust if you are flying from west to east, as in this example.

For your London flight, start five or six days ahead of departure and back off your normal sleeping time by an hour or so each day. This means that, on the day before your flight, you are probably going to bed at a very early hour—six or seven in the evening. But when you arrive, you will be mostly adjusted. Life being what it is, you could settle for an 8 P.M. bedtime by the time you leave and do fairly well.

A basic rule for beating jet lag is very simple, whether you are going east or west. That is to immediately adapt to the local living patterns, rhythms, and times, rather than trying to keep to your own. When everyone else is eating dinner, you do the same. When they all retire for the evening, do the same. When they get up, you do the same. You may experience periods of drowsiness during the day or wakefulness in the evening, especially at first, but your body will get the message.

It's important to pay attention during the flight as well. Alcohol is probably not a good idea, nor is it a good idea to stuff yourself with those delicious airline dinners, even if you are fortunate enough to be flying in first class. Airplane air is dry, dry, dry. Drink bottled water and eat lightly. Try not to doze off if you're heading west, although that might be the right thing to do if you're going east. It depends on the time changes—when you started and what time it will be when you get there. Heavy carbohydrates are a no-no—you could go for the chicken Caesar (if there's a choice) or even bring food with you that has a high protein content.

If you are going east, get out in the light as much as you can once you're there. Remember, your best shot at defeating jet lag is taking the trouble to prepare yourself ahead of time by making the effort to adjust your internal rhythms. It's worth it in terms of enjoyment and alertness when you reach your destination.

Jet Lag Checklist

Here's a list of do's and don'ts for beating jet lag. Do the best you can to meet the suggestions on the list, but don't make yourself crazy about it. Most of these are commonsense things that you might normally be doing if you were in your own time zone, but take into consideration that the time frame is different where you are going. Don't get carried away if you are only going from New York to Chicago. But if it's one of those mind twisters across half the world, take a good look at this list.

—— Drink lots of water on the plane and avoid alcohol.

—— If you are going west to east, catch a few Z's on the plane, if you can.

—— If you are going east to west, try to stay awake, or limit your nap to about forty-five minutes.

—— Try to schedule your flight for afternoon or early evening arrival. Avoid putting yourself in one of those situations where you dash to the hotel and then into downtown Jakarta, or wherever, for an important meeting.

—— Try using 0.3 to 0.5 milligrams of melatonin to trigger sleep on the plane (west to east) about two hours before you want to sleep. (See chapter 5 for more on melatonin.)

—— Keep cool. If it's one of those flights where someone cranked up the heat, ask the flight attendant to adjust it. Don't wimp out; ask again if doesn't get handled in a reasonable period of time. When you get to your destination, set the temperature in your room at a cool level. When you are sleeping, your body temperature drops by as much as two degrees—temperature is one of the triggers for sleep.

—— Immediately adapt to the time frame and rhythms of the time zone. Eat, sleep, work, and play when everyone else is doing the same. Take it easy on the local cuisine at first—your digestive system needs to adjust. You can try using a small dose of melatonin to trigger sleep if you have to, one to two hours before bedtime.

—— Get out in the light when you get up—turn everything on, throw open the curtains, step out onto the balcony. More light is better.

—— Exercise on the plane. That doesn't mean push-ups in the aisle, but you can walk up and down, stretch, or do isometrics. Be creative and make up your own routine. Don't stay planted in your seat for the whole trip. If nothing else, the typical airline seat is guaranteed to drive you into the aisle sooner or later—make the most of it.

—— Do a few simple exercises or stretches in the morning when you get up.

—— Don't drink coffee or caffeinated soft drinks on the plane, especially if it's going to be nighttime when you arrive. Coffee and other caffeine drinks will dehydrate your body, so if you do indulge, follow it up with lots of water. On the other hand, a little green tea might refresh your soul in a way that is more than worth the small intake of caffeine that goes with it. Or take the teas you like with you for the trip.

—— Anything you can do to entertain yourself and keep your body and mind occupied is a good idea.

I have one more trick for jet lag, but you may think it's pretty strange, and in fact it is. It doesn't always work, and it requires a developed ability to calm yourself and visualize internally. When it does work, it's amazing, and I am the first to say that I don't really understand why. It is a kind of meditation geared toward getting your body to adjust to the disruption caused by relocating yourself halfway around the world in a matter of hours. I discovered it on a long flight to India.

The idea behind the trick is this: while you are zooming through the air at forty thousand feet and at several hundred miles an hour, some part of you is still hanging out back in your home time zone. That is why people refer to the whole problem as jet lag—it feels as if this is what's happening. If that were actually true, then it would make sense to try to get the part that is lagging behind to catch up with you. This ought to make you feel better. The reason is that this part that got left behind might be the part that needs to catch up over time (about an hour a day) in your new time zone.

See, I told you it was strange. Obviously this can't possibly have anything to do with the physiology of the internal clock and all the rest of it, unless it somehow creates an instant resetting of the clock in a way that can't really be understood. Perhaps I thought this up as the result of not having enough to do on long flights, but wherever it came from, it can actually work. If it works you will not have to go through jet lag, or the effects will at least be greatly moderated. I speak from experience. Here's the technique—take it for what it's worth.

A Jet Lag Trick to Catch Up to Yourself

—— Wait until you are at least halfway to your destination before you begin this visualization. Don't do it when you are likely to be interrupted by food service or some other routine event. Don't do it right after food service, when your seatmate is likely to want to make a bathroom run. Wait until all is calm. It can be done during a movie, if you like, unless you want to watch the show.

—— Get yourself as comfortable as possible in your seat, take a few deep breaths, and close your eyes. It helps to have a tape recorder with earphones and a pleasant and relaxing musical tape playing during the visualization.

—— With your eyes closed, continue to breathe easily and deeply. Allow yourself to become very aware of your body, how it feels, the physical sensations, the noises of the engines and the feeling of the cabin around you—in short, get totally present in a conscious, relaxed and focused way. We often try to shut out all of the annoying things in the airplane experience. The key to this exercise is inclusion rather than pushing away. I'll say it again: the key is inclusion, not exclusion of everything that is happening in the plane.

—— Continue to breathe easily and let your awareness of the plane fade naturally. You are not shutting it out; rather, as you begin to focus, the result is a natural fading of distractions.

—— Focus your attention on the center of your chest and back. By "focus your attention" I mean that you imagine and feel yourself as thinking and experiencing everything in the center of your chest and back. Imagine that you can hear, feel, think, etc., in the center of your body. Bring your entire awareness to the middle of your body, right behind your breastbone. Let this feeling develop. You can actually "think" in any part of your body, so let yourself think in the center of your chest.

—— Now visualize the airport that you left behind at the beginning of your trip. In your mind's eye, see yourself in the airport. Make it seem real. Imagine that somehow you are actually still there in the airport, if not in body, then in some other way—as if part of you got left behind. Keep yourself focused in the center of your chest.

—— Imagine that there is a connection of some sort between you in the seat of the airplane and that part which got left behind in the airport when you flew away. Think of it like some kind of tenuous substance or perhaps like a thin band of something stretching all the way back from your seat to the airport. See it stretching back, in your mind's eye, back through the clouds and the sky, back over the water and the land, all the way back to the airport. Feel it. Make it real. As you are rushing forward in the airplane, the connection stretches away behind you.

—— Now, imagine that you can pull that part which was left behind in the airport to you. Just as if it was at the end of a long rubber band, imagine this part lifting away from the airport and somehow being able to come to where you are in the airplane, following along that thin band you have visualized in your mind's eye. Pull it to you.

—— You may suddenly feel as if something has actually snapped forward along the imaginary connection and collided with you, striking you somewhere in the back. It could simply be a gentle sense of something melding back together within you. It could be that you will get no sensation at all. Whatever you get, relax and give it a chance to happen.

—— When you feel that the exercise is complete, take a breath and open your eyes.

It's possible for this exercise to eliminate any effects of jet lag. When you get off the plane, you will be almost perfectly adjusted to the local time. This is a claim that is absolutely unprovable in a scientific sense, but it can be a reality you experience, and that is what matters. I'm practically oriented, and I want results. To me, the experience feels as though something suddenly zooms along the imaginary connection trailing behind me and comes back into my physical body. I immediately feel better. Yes, it's very weird, but it really does work sometimes. You won't know unless you try it. At the very least you will have managed to pass a little more of the time on your long flight, and your body will benefit from the relaxed breathing and calm mind. Good luck with it.

YOU ARE IN CHARGE

We can find a lot of reasons for losing sleep if we want to. A special occasion, pressures in our work situation, squeezing in extra activities in a busy life, the needs of family and children— the list is almost endless. It's okay to lose some sleep once in a while, and we all do it when we have something that seems more important to us. But when we lose sleep consistently, it's a different story entirely. If we were actually prevented from sleeping at all, we would eventually die. Preventing a prisoner from sleeping has long been a method of torture in places where human rights are not respected.

When someone is deprived completely of sleep, a strange thing happens. After enough time has passed, over a period of days, something goes wrong with the temperature regulation in the body. The victim can no longer maintain the necessary body heat and becomes colder and colder and then dies. This has been documented by Amnesty International in the tales of survivors who have escaped repressive regimes in Latin America.

It's likely that none of us will ever find ourselves in such a terrible situation, but there are plenty of ill effects that follow if we continually miss out on the sleep we need. Depression, irritability, bad decision making, loss of memory, ruined relationships, physical illness, dangerous behaviors, and poor judgment are just a few, certain results. There's a real risk of physical injury, and even death, because of sleep-deprived actions and decisions.

Sleep Well, Sleep Deep

If you are one of the seventy or eighty million Americans who cannot sleep well on any given night, there's a lot you can do to bring normal sleep back into your life. Like any other change in life habits, it requires conscious attention and a desire to get a different result. It requires more than wishful thinking, but the good news is that in most cases it doesn't take a long time to get the benefit of better sleep or to make the kinds of changes that may be necessary. Sometimes there is a physical reason for sleeplessness that needs to be addressed by a physician. Often it's simply a matter of taking a look at the habits and patterns of living that mark the rhythms of your life, making some simple changes and moving on. In the next chapter we'll look at some of the things you can do when you can't sleep.

CHAPTER TWO

WHAT TO DO WHEN YOU CAN'T SLEEP

It's two o'clock in the morning. You've been trying to get to sleep for several hours, and your bed feels like something from that camping trip you took when you were ten years old. You're tossing and turning. What can you do to get to sleep?

For a lasting fix, we'll have to find out what you might have done to avoid sleeplessness in the first place. Later on in this chapter there is a simple "sleep potential" inventory that helps identify many common causes of sleeplessness. Acting on the information revealed by the inventory lets you take charge of your sleeping life. But before we get to that, here are a few simple ideas that can help you ease off into dreamland.

—— One of the simplest things that helps is often overlooked: get up and get out of bed if you've been lying there awake for twenty minutes or more. Once you've been awake that long, it's best to let the sheets cool down and give your body a break from trying to relax.

—— Put on a robe or whatever makes you feel comfortable, get out of the bedroom, and go sit in a comfortable chair in the dark. Yes, in the dark, because if you turn on the lights you run the risk of tricking the brain into thinking it's time to get up and get going; that's not what you want to do. A recliner is perfect, because you can almost lie down, and recliners tend to be comfortable chairs. If you don't have a recliner, a couch or soft chair will do fine. Don't turn on the television! The light from the screen and the programming tend to overstimulate the cerebral cortex and make it harder to sleep. After about twenty minutes to a half-hour, go back to bed and get comfortable. This may be enough to let you get to sleep. If not, there are other things you can do.

—— Sometimes you can take two aspirin if you can't sleep. After about a half-hour it kicks in and acts like a mild relaxant. If you are allergic to aspirin, Tylenol or another substitute will work as well. The idea is to help you relax on a deeper, physical level, without resorting to sleeping pills or some other strong medication. Many of us carry subconscious levels of muscular stress and tension, below the threshold of pain but quite susceptible to the light "hit" of a mild analgesic like aspirin. Getting that stress to release will help you sleep. Some research contradicts this advice, but I have always found it effective. Experiment, and let your results be your guide. Everyone is a little different.

—— A technique that works well for some people involves inner visualization. The jet lag trick in the last chapter is an example of visualization. If you are able to clearly see something in your mind's eye (some of us have trouble visualizing), then this might be the right approach for you. It works like this: as you are lying in bed realizing that you are having trouble getting to sleep, think of something that feels inspirational or peaceful and calming to you. It could be an actual memory of a real place or it could be something you create with your imagination. For example, you might imagine that you are standing in a beautiful mountain meadow on a clear, sunny day. In your mind's eye, see the flowers, the sky and clouds, the mountains, and any other details you can imagine. Let yourself create the picture in your mind and then feel it as if it were real. Focus your attention on the calm beauty of the scene. When you succeed in doing this, you will fall asleep. It's like magic, like creating your own instant dream. Pick a place and a setting that feels calming and peaceful to you.

One major cause of sleeplessness is a busy mind. It's as if something inside us simply won't be quiet, insists that we look at something, think about something, figure something out, or solve some problem. It can be like a waking nightmare. If you are overly tired or highly stressed about work or some other situation, a busy mind is a common result.

The way to calm a busy mind is to give it something else to do that will help you sleep. That way the mind is still doing what it thinks it's supposed to do (be busy), but you are using the busyness to get yourself to sleep. This is the reasoning behind the old "counting sheep" trick that you have probably heard about. In this classic, you imagine sheep jumping over a fence and count them as they go by, until you fall asleep. The only problem is that today, many of us haven't got a clue about what a sheep is really like, and we are liable to conjure up some kind of vague or fuzzy four-legged animal in our mind's eye, if we can see it at all. Sheep as an image doesn't really speak to most of us the way it may have in the rural past of our ancestors. Pick something familiar to count. It could be anything from toasters to basketballs.

——— A variation on this approach is to imagine numbers against a black background. Start at 100 and visualize your hand placing the number in gold against the black. You can use other colors, if you prefer—it's up to you. Once you have managed to clearly imagine the number 100, you take it down and put up 99. You continue in this way, counting backward and waiting until each number is clearly seen against the background before you go on to the next. I'd be very surprised if you ever make it to zero before falling asleep. Your busy mind will be very happy to assist you with this task, as the part that is "busy" doesn't really care what it's busy about, so long as it has something to do.

A trick that works for some people who play golf or another sport is to go back over your last game. As you replay it shot by shot, hole by hole, you fall asleep. This could backfire if you begin analyzing what you did wrong (or right) during the game.

——— Sometimes you can make a deal with the busy mind, but this takes practice. The deal usually goes something like this: in an internal dialogue, promise yourself that you will definitely address whatever the problem is tomorrow, after you get some sleep, if in return your mind will quiet down and allow sleep to come. Sound silly? Believe me, this can work. But be warned—you must indeed do what you promised yourself you would do. Otherwise, your mind will be back the next time you are trying to sleep, busier than ever, with an added agenda of making sure you realize that you have double-crossed yourself.

——— Often people like to use music to fall asleep, but I personally am wary of this approach, because I believe they are conditioning themselves to sleep only when they hear the music. This can be a problem if, for some reason, the music isn't available. If you must use something, I suggest a recording of nature, especially of the ocean. There is an excellent CD available called *Solitudes* (Vol. 2, *The Sound of the Surf*) that features superb ocean recordings. Play this gently in the background, and the sound of the waves breaking on a distant shore can lull you to relaxation and sleep. There are also "white noise" machines on the market that can serve the same purpose.

A sure prescription for sleep is getting the body and mind to relax, to let go and feel at ease. Anything we can do to promote ease and relaxation will help. One simple, effective technique that can help you get to sleep is focusing on your breathing. I have used different breathing techniques for different purposes over many years, and I've found they are powerful tools for accomplishing whatever particular goal is desired, like getting to sleep.

Most breathing techniques and patterns that regulate the mind and body have their roots in ancient India, in Ayurvedic teachings that include yoga and other mind/body/spirit disciplines. Thousands of years of practice have confirmed their worth, if properly practiced and applied. Dr. Andrew Weil, the author of several successful books on health and well-being, has popularized one particular breathing technique.

Begin by placing the tip of your tongue on the roof of your mouth, just in back of your front teeth. Keep the tongue lightly touching behind the teeth throughout the entire sequence. This initiates a pathway of subtle energy (according to the ancient teachings) and has a healing, calming, and restorative effect.

Inhale deeply through your nose to a count of four; hold the breath for a count of seven; and then release the breath through your mouth with a soft whooshing sound for a count of eight. As you do so, simply pay attention to the breath as it enters and leaves your body. Don't get hung up on how long or how deep your breath is, but aim for consistency in the count, so that all beats fall to the same rhythm. Do this for a cycle of four times. At the end of the cycle, if you have done it correctly, you will notice that you feel calmer, more centered and more relaxed in your body. This is also a quietly energizing breath you can use during the day or in the morning. At night, you can use it to still the chatter of your mind and ease your body back toward slumber. You may find it more comfortable to sit up when you do this exercise.

—— Hunger can awaken you or keep you awake, so if that is the problem, you should eat something. Remember to be conscious about it. Don't eat things like ice cream, chocolate, or anything with a high sugar content. That will keep you awake. Don't stuff yourself. Don't be like Dagwood in the comics, who raids the refrigerator in the middle of the night and makes himself an arm-length sandwich. Eat something light and mildly filling. Popcorn might work, but the noise of making it and chewing it might not. Maybe a bowl of soup, or even the traditional glass of warm milk, if you like milk.

—— Self-hypnosis can help you relax and fall asleep. There is an entire chapter devoted to self-hypnosis later in the book, so I will not cover that here. Follow the directions given there and you will most likely have good success.

It's necessary to experiment with different approaches to find what works for you most of the time. It may take a combination of things, and it may take practice, but if you persevere you will be well on your way to taking charge of your sleep.

Taking charge of sleep is like any other self-improvement idea we want to adopt. It requires thought and action. Each one of us has our own unique situation. Developing a strategy for better sleep requires thinking it through and taking particular needs, preferences, and personal quirks into account. Action is required: just as in exercise programs or dietary changes, it takes specific, concrete steps to make change happen. Thinking about it without doing something about it doesn't bring any results.

Before we make an overall plan for improving our rest, we have to discover what is really disrupting our sleep. Would you like to find out right now what might be affecting yours? You may be surprised at how many different things can adversely influence our sleep.

Below is a personal inventory of habits and other elements that can affect sleep. It consists of a series of statements, with four possible responses to each one. You can use this to measure your "sleep potential." There is no correct response to any statement. You simply want to get a good picture of the factors in your life affecting sleep and perhaps contributing to poor sleep and restless nights. The inventory is an easy, quick way to get the information you need. Just circle the response that seems closest to your particular situation, and we'll consider what it all means afterward. Don't take it too seriously—have fun!

PERSONAL SLEEP INVENTORY: WHAT'S YOUR SLEEP POTENTIAL?

1. I usually go to bed at about the same time each night, and get up at about the same time each morning.
   a. Always
   b. Almost always
   c. Rarely
   d. Never

2. My bed is very comfortable.
  a. Yes, it is.
  b. It's pretty good; it mostly feels comfortable to me.
  c. It's not so hot, but it's a bed.
  d. It's like sleeping on lumps of coal.

3. My bedroom is always quiet.
  a. It always is, at least when I'm going to sleep and during the night.
  b. Usually it is, but sometimes there are noises.
  c. There can be a lot of noise at night, depending on what's going on.
  d. About as quiet as a subway train.

4. Alcohol helps me go to sleep.
  a. I don't drink before bed or to help me sleep.
  b. A drink in the early evening helps me relax from the day.
  c. I think a drink before bedtime relaxes me and helps me sleep.
  d. I have a hard time getting to sleep unless I have a drink or two before bed.

5. I have a lot of pain in my body.
  a. No, I'm lucky not to have any.
  b. Not very much—an aspirin will handle it when necessary.
  c. Sometimes it's hard to sleep because I'm so uncomfortable.
  d. I have pain all the time, and sometimes it's pretty severe.

6. I like to have a bedtime snack.
  a. No, it's unusual for me to eat right before bed.
  b. Sometimes I snack before bed, but not often.
  c. I usually eat something not long before bed.
  d. I love to eat before bed—I get hungry and I feel better if I eat something.

7. I usually wake up in the middle of the night and go to the bathroom.
- **a.** Never, I just sleep through.
- **b.** Sometimes I get up, but not very often.
- **c.** I usually have to get up.
- **d.** I always get up—doesn't everybody?

8. I feel relaxed and at ease most of the time.
- **a.** Yes, life's pretty easy.
- **b.** Well, mostly I do, but things get to me sometimes.
- **c.** I'm not sure anymore what it means to be relaxed.
- **d.** I'm always worried and tensed up about something.

9. I've been told that I snore a lot, and loudly, too.
- **a.** Not me, I sleep like a baby.
- **b.** Sometimes I guess I snore when I'm tired.
- **c.** Yes, I have been told that.
- **d.** I snore all the time, and it shakes the roof.

10. My legs get twitchy and jumpy when I'm asleep.
- **a.** Never.
- **b.** I move around some.
- **c.** Sometimes I wake up because my legs jump.
- **d.** Every night you'd think I was running the marathon.

11. I get enough exercise to feel good about myself and my health.
- **a.** That describes me perfectly.
- **b.** I get some exercise several times a week.
- **c.** Every once in a while I go for a walk.
- **d.** I never exercise if I can avoid it.

12. The temperature in my bedroom is just right.
   a. I'm always comfortable.
   b. It varies some, but it's not a problem.
   c. Often it seems too hot or too cold.
   d. It never seems right.

13. I like to work, read, and think things through in bed.
   a. I think beds are best left to romance and sleeping.
   b. Once in a while I'll read a book in bed.
   c. I like to hang out in bed and read or think.
   d. That's a good place to get some work done.

14. I get sleepy during the day.
   a. No, I always feel alert.
   b. Sometimes I get a little sleepy after lunch.
   c. I feel as if I really need to take a nap during the afternoon.
   d. I have to fight to stay alert all during the day.

15. I have a medical condition that can wake me up at night.
   a. No, I'm healthy as a horse.
   b. Sometimes I'll catch something that makes it hard to sleep.
   c. Yes, but I have it under control and usually I can sleep.
   d. I have to wake up a lot to deal with it.

16. I like to drink a lot of coffee during the day.
   a. I don't drink coffee.
   b. I have a cup in the morning and sometimes one in the afternoon.
   c. I usually drink about a pot during the course of the day.
   d. I couldn't keep going if I didn't drink a lot of coffee, and I like a cup after dinner.

17. I smoke, and I usually have a cigarette before bed.
  a. I don't smoke at all.
  b. I quit a while ago, but I still have an occasional cigarette.
  c. I smoke some, but usually not right before bed.
  d. I really enjoy that last cigarette of the day.

18. My work schedule is regular and consistent, with the same hours every day.
  a. Sure, I'm in control of my schedule and I keep it consistent.
  b. Usually, but sometimes I have to work longer than I want to.
  c. My schedule rotates on different shifts each week, but it's consistent.
  d. I work when they want me to, or when I have to, because of the job.

19. I travel a lot in my work and often stay overnight.
  a. I never have to go anywhere, unless it's for a vacation.
  b. Sometimes I have to travel.
  c. I travel a lot, but I'm able to get home for several days each week.
  d. I have to travel all the time, and I'm lucky if I make it home for the weekend.

20. My mind is usually calm when I'm lying in bed getting ready to sleep.
  a. Yes, that's one thing I like about going to bed.
  b. Mostly, but sometimes it takes a while to settle down.
  c. A lot of times it's hard to stop thinking about things, but I usually drift off after a while.
  d. If I don't force myself to stop thinking so much about everything, I can't sleep.

Sleep Well, Sleep Deep

Here's how to score your responses and get a quick snapshot of your sleep potential. Get a sheet of paper, and give yourself a 5 for every **a** response, a 4 for every **b** response, a 3 for every **c**, and a 2 for every **d**. Add them up. By the way, if you answered **a** to every statement, congratulations! You get 100, probably have no problems sleeping, and may wonder why you are reading this book.

A "perfect" score for measuring your sleep potential would be 100 (20 questions × 5 = 100). A score of 40 (20 questions × 2 = 40) would be the most disturbing result, because that would indicate that you have both medical problems that need to be addressed and a sleeping environment that is utterly miserable. I hope none of you scored this low, but if you did, you would be wise to seek out professional help right away. Some sleep resources are given at the end of the book. Almost all of us will fall somewhere between these two extremes.

A score of 80 or better is excellent, in terms of your sleep potential. There are a few things you can do to make a difference and improve your sleep. A score between 65 and 80 shows there is real room for improvement and is an average score—remember, seventy to eighty million people have trouble sleeping in our country on any given night. A score of 50 to 65 indicates that you have a genuine sleeping problem. You can probably get some very fast benefits by making some adjustments, but you have some serious thinking to do and may need medical or other professional advice if you want to get more sleep. And finally, anything below 50 is a signal to pay immediate attention.

A low score indicates you are very likely sleep-deprived. That can lead to errors of judgment, health problems, poor decision making, and all of the other results of habitual loss of sleep. The good news is that you are the one who is in charge; you are the one who can shift the balance to better sleep and rest, if you want to badly enough.

Contained in this brief inventory are many of the common factors making for bad sleep and worse rest. Mental stress and worry, physical pain, addictions to alcohol or other drugs (including nicotine, caffeine, and some prescription drugs) will keep sleep away. An exhaustive work schedule, shift work that breaks up the regular day/night rhythms, a crummy bed, or a noisy and otherwise unsatisfactory sleep environment will do it. Disturbances during the night (like pets jumping on the bed or children crying), drinking too much liquid before bed (full bladder), or eating too much before bed are all sleep destroyers. Medical factors (such as allergies, asthma, stomach and digestive problems, sleep disorders), excessive naps during the day, not enough exercise—all these things, and more, can make sleep elusive or impossible.

If a particular statement hits home, then you can certainly do something about what is revealed and get a good result! It's up to you. By looking at each statement in turn we can see how the topic affects sleep for better or worse and devise a strategy for dealing with it, if necessary.

1. I usually go to bed at about the same time each night, and get up at about the same time each morning.

This statement reflects the reality of the circadian body rhythms talked about in chapter 1. Your body likes routine and regularity, especially when it comes to sleeping. There is a name for what happens when things get out of step: "delayed sleep phase syndrome." This is when your sleeping hours are out of rhythm and your internal body clock resets itself to a new cycle and a new, later bedtime. It's fine to be out late on the weekend and enjoy yourself, but if you make it a habit to stay up late, you run the risk of resetting the clock. Then, when you have to get up for the old workday shuffle, you are groggy, tired, and subject to all the symptoms of not enough sleep. Worse, when you decide enough is enough and attempt to go to bed at a reasonable time, you find that you can't get to sleep.

The solution is simple: make it a habit to go to bed at about the same time each night, and make sure that your chosen time provides enough for approximately eight hours of sleep before you have to get up and get ready for your day.

Not so long ago many researchers believed that eight hours of sleep was too much and that most people could get along just fine on five hours a night. But in fact, only about two percent of us function well on this kind of sleep cycle. Unless you are among this two percent, you will not be at your best with much less than the eight hours that fit your natural rhythm. Seven and a half to eight and a half hours are ideal for almost all of us.

If you think that you will have difficulty fitting eight hours of sleep into your life, then it might not be a bad idea to take a look at your priorities. If you are not sleeping well, then sleep really should become your priority, no matter what protest your mind makes about it. And protest it will, because if you are not already set up for an eight-hour sleep cycle, there must be a good "reason" for it, like work or play.

If you have been on a cycle that gets you to bed too late for enough sleep before you have to get up, then you need to make the adjustment. It's much better to change your pattern than it is to try to catch up when you can, either by sleeping in on some days or taking naps during the day. Unfortunately, we can't store sleep and pull out its restorative power when we need it. If we could, it would be a lot easier.

2. My bed is very comfortable.

This one sounds like a no-brainer, since it makes sense that a good bed will contribute to a good night's rest. The only problem is that there are a lot of ideas about what exactly constitutes a "good" bed. The issue is further complicated because one person's idea of a good bed may be something just this short of cement, while his or her partner or spouse may think that something a little softer than marshmallows is about right.

That brings up a key issue: the differences between us, revealed in our subjective feelings about what is good and what is not. There are umpteen television ads that reflect that truth. For example, one of those ads touts a bed that keeps movement on one side away from the person sleeping on the other. Is that a good bed? Only you can tell, and only by lying down on it in a way that actually tests the comfort levels. What is certain is that if you and your partner have different subjective preferences about sleep, bedtimes, mattresses, and other common factors that affect sleep, there may be a problem. The solution is usually to talk it through and find a mutually satisfactory compromise.

In general, better beds cost more, a fact which is sad but true. That $300 king size special you see in the Sunday paper may look attractive, but it will have some serious shortfalls when it comes to durability and long-term comfort. That is partially because cheaper mattresses have fewer coils to support the body. More coils equal better support. Each manufacturer may have a different system for tying those coils together, and that also makes a difference.

On the other hand, you don't necessarily have to pay $1,500 for a good bed, either. Bells and whistles have been added to most major lines to make the bed appear attractive, special, and elite. Like car tires, beds come with warranties for years of use, but I suspect it's harder to measure the wear.

The decision about whether a bed is comfortable or not is purely subjective. Try it out and be selective. In the meantime, if you circled **c** or **d** on this question, seriously consider getting a new bed. You'll be glad you did.

3. My bedroom is always quiet.

A noisy sleep environment is one of the worst villains for ruining sleep. If you are lucky enough to have a quiet bedroom, then this isn't a factor you need to consider. Many people, however, live in environments where noise is more or less constant. Even a slight noise can disturb sleep; this is true whether or not you actually become fully or consciously awake.

Apartments are great offenders in this area, because of course you can't control what happens on either side of or above you. There's nothing like having someone lifting weights above your ceiling at three in the morning! One strategy if you have a noisy apartment is to do something to deaden and absorb sounds. Rugs are great for this, as is heavy furniture like couches and sofas. Hang colorful rugs on the walls and you will not only get comments about your decorating skills but will also lessen the sound transmitted through those walls and reflected into the apartment. Put drapes on the windows if you can and if you like them. Open windows are a problem, especially in the city. Sometimes it's a tradeoff between cooler temperatures and excessive noise. Temperature will usually win.

You can always try earplugs. I like the ones made of soft foam that expand to block your ears. (I hate the wax kind, which feel slimy and wet to me.) A box with several sets of plugs can be found in your local supermarket or pharmacy for around three dollars. Earplugs really help if you have a sleeping partner who snores.

A better approach for noise control may be to set up a constant background of "white noise" to mask the offending sounds from outside. Some people react well to this, others do not. White noise is nonspecific background noise at a steady level. I prefer a recording of ocean waves to the constant type. There are also simple devices on the market that provide the sound desired.

Be creative, and try your best to create a quiet sleep environment—it's worth the effort.

4. Alcohol helps me go to sleep.

One of the most pervasive myths of sleep is that having a "nightcap" will help you sleep. It's true that if you have a drink or two and are tired you may go to sleep very quickly when you lie down. That is the basis for the myth, along with the idea that alcohol helps many people to relax. It's not that simple, because going to sleep initially is only a small part of getting a good night's rest.

Alcohol is a depressant. It interrupts the normal functioning of the nervous system. When it wears off, the result is increased wakefulness (although not alertness), irritability, and a tendency to disrupt the normal REM cycle of sleeping. In other words, when you drink, you will tend to wake up in an hour or two feeling unrested and having trouble getting back to sleep. When you wake in the morning, you may also have consequences, including headache, tiredness, jumpiness, and a general sense of dullness. I'm not talking about the classic hangover that comes from over-indulgence—just the reality of using alcohol to help you sleep.

Many alcoholics got started because they had trouble sleeping and decided that a good stiff shot of something helped them get to sleep. Alcohol is a powerful and addictive drug, and it needs to be treated as such. I am not against drinking socially, and I like a glass or two now and then. But before bedtime it's a certain setup for bad sleep. The older you are, the longer the stretch of time before bed when you should avoid drinking. The absolute minimum is about two hours. For me, that's too close.

Don't drink to get to sleep. If you have a great deal of trouble relaxing or if you drink to dull pain, you may want to consider seeing a physician. That glass of cognac or whisky may knock you out at first, but later you may feel just like a boxer coming to in the locker room. Your body will give you cause for regret.

5. I have a lot of pain in my body.

This is a tough one, because pain isn't something you can make go away with white noise or a better mattress. Unfortunately, many people suffer chronic pain, sometimes very severe pain.

If you have a medical condition or disease process that causes severe pain, I hope you are under the care of a physician. There are various drugs that alleviate pain. There is a problem with some of them, because they can be disruptive to sleep. In general, the least amount of a pain medication that will help is the best amount. It's all too easy to overdo it. If you are taking medication for pain that interferes with sleep, talk with your doctor and see if there is an alternative.

If I had the answer to the mastery of pain, many people would probably hail me as a savior. I don't have that answer. However, there is a trick or two that can assist you in handling pain and reducing its effect.

Of course the first thing is to identify and understand the cause of the pain. It's one thing if you are simply stiff and sore from a hard day's work; it's another if there is a medical cause. Assuming that you have identified the cause, the next step is to lessen the feeling.

There are basically three ways that I know of to work with pain. The first is medication. For example, narcotics act within the brain to deaden sensation. The problem here is that they are addictive and have other consequences. If you are taking strong pain medication and this is interfering with your sleep, talk with your doctor about it. No self-help book can adequately address this beyond suggesting that there may be alternatives for you to explore. I'll leave the issue of prescription medication for pain to you and your doctor.

The second method for controlling pain involves direct application of physical techniques to the body. In this category are things like warm baths, hot and cold applications, exercise (*e.g.*, yoga), and massage. You can choose any of these and get good results, depending on your situation and the nature of the pain. Yoga and exercise can act to prevent pain before it starts. Some yoga is designed to specifically relieve joint pain, for example. If you are sore, particularly if you have muscular soreness, then the other suggestions can work well to alleviate the pain.

The third approach is perhaps the most difficult but also the most rewarding, because it puts you directly in charge on a very fundamental level. This approach uses the mind to work with pain, with the result that the pain lessens or disappears. Sound impossible? You can learn to make pain bearable or even to go away.

Of course, I am assuming that you are not going to use these techniques without an understanding of the root cause of the pain. That could lead to trouble. For example, suppose you succeed in making chronic headache pain disappear. That's great in terms of immediate relief, but what if it is a brain tumor that is causing the pain? If you eliminate the symptom without investigating the cause, you run the risk of harming yourself. Be responsible about the way you feel in your body. In particular, chronic pain is a warning sign that should be heeded. Chronic pain is a good reason to think about seeing a physician, to determine if the cause requires medical treatment.

Having said that, the first principle of controlling pain with the mind is this: we must become attuned to the pain before we can make it go away. This means we have to allow ourselves to fully experience the pain before we can work with it, a radically different way of dealing with pain. What we usually do is try to push the pain away or ignore it. (Remember, I did say this was a difficult approach.)

Something odd happens when we succeed in fully surrendering to pain: it becomes less. Just the act of not resisting the sensation, as difficult as it sounds, can make the sensation disappear. Allowing yourself to fully surrender to pain is not a common perspective; it's not the way we usually think. Once we have admitted to ourselves that something hurts like blazes, we can get on to the next steps of managing the hurt.

Once we attune and accept the pain in this way, we have a couple of choices about how to proceed. We can use self-hypnosis, or we can use techniques of inner visualization to handle the pain. Self-hypnosis will be discussed later on in the book. Inner visualization is different.

For example, suppose you have a really bad headache. Nothing has worked, and your head is splitting. You lie in bed, unable to sleep, head pounding and wishing you could just make it go away. Years ago I learned a simple visualization that is very effective—I think it was created by Werner Erhard, but it may be older. With your eyes closed, describe the headache to yourself in specific detail and tune in to it, seeing it in your mind's eye. What color is it? What shape? Where is it located exactly? On a scale of one to ten (ten being highest), how intense is it? Ask yourself these questions and note the answer. Then repeat the process. You will find that the answers change. The color, the shape, the location, and, finally, the intensity will change, if you really tune in and focus on the headache in this way. You may start with an "eight" and then quickly realize that the pain has reduced to a "five" or a "four." Continue in this way until the headache is gone or barely noticeable.

You can do the same with any pain, anywhere in your body. It does take practice. It's true also that really severe pain can be so overwhelming that you literally cannot think straight, making this kind of visualization technique next to impossible. In that case, wait until a time when the pain is bearable or absent. Learn the self-hypnosis techniques given later and apply them the next time pain strikes. What have you got to lose by trying? Only the pain.

Pain is a signal from some part of the body that something needs attention. Before the brain can register the pain signal and respond (with pain), the signal must travel along the nerves and the spinal cord and enter the brain. Sometimes we can do something to distract ourselves or interrupt the signal in some way, so that the sensation of pain is dulled or disappears.

A physician may recommend a TENS (transcutaneous electrical nerve stimulator) device. This instrument delivers a tiny electrical shock to the affected area, on demand. The electrical impulses stimulate many nerve endings and overwhelm the pain signals being transmitted; the result is a lessening or relief of pain. I have used one of these, and they do work. You can get the same effect by using a stiff hairbrush and stroking the affected area. That triggers the nerve endings and blocks the pain signal.

Whatever you do, the thing to remember is this: you *can* control most kinds of pain, and you can manage pain so that it does not interfere with your sleep. Don't give up.

6. I like to have a bedtime snack.

If your response was **c** or **d** to this statement, eating may be affecting your sleep. It's okay to have a light snack before bed if you are especially hungry, as might be the case several hours after dinner. A light snack is one thing, but a meal is another.

Asking the digestive system to handle a large pizza before bed, for example, is definitely not recommended. Your body gets mixed messages. Because you are lying down you run an increased risk of acid moving up the esophagus and other unpleasant effects. Your system tries to digest but is basically in the wrong gravitational relationship for good digestion and has to work a lot harder. The result is interrupted sleep.

The solution is easy. Avoid heavy foods or large amounts of food before you go to bed. Simple!

7. I usually wake up in the middle of the night and go to the bathroom.

Unless there is a medical reason, most of us shouldn't have to get up often during the night to relieve a full bladder. Getting up disturbs our rest, plus it's no fun stumbling around in the dark.

If you have small children, you know that a basic rule of thumb is to keep drinks away from them after a certain hour, as they approach bedtime. A sip is fine, but a glass of water is not. Forget this and you may have a wet bed to deal with the next day or in the middle of the night. It's just simple physiology: the only difference between you and the children is that you have a larger capacity to store fluids, and you are also "trained" to wake up and go to the bathroom if you have to.

Like the children, the solution is to avoid drinking a lot before bedtime. Pretty basic, but we forget that simple things like this make a difference. By the way, too much alcohol will dehydrate the body, causing you to wake in the night needing a drink of water, with perhaps a consequent trip to the bathroom before dawn.

If you have to get up frequently to urinate during the night, this may be a sign of a physical problem that needs to be addressed. For example, frequent urination is one of the signs of prostate enlargement in men. Other medical conditions can cause this symptom as well, such as blood-sugar problems. At the risk of sounding like a broken record, this might be a good reason to consult a physician. Sleep is such a key part of our health and well-being that any serious disruption in our sleeping life may be a reflection of an underlying health problem.

8. I feel relaxed and at ease most of the time.

Most of us carry a lot of tension. Life can be very stressful and worrisome. There are many techniques for relaxation and stress relief, as the self-help section of any bookstore will quickly demonstrate. This statement is in the sleep inventory to remind you that relaxation is crucial to good sleep and rest. As we go further into the list of statements, it becomes apparent that there are many interrelationships that can affect sleep. For example, it's hard to relax if you are in pain, so pain relief becomes a precursor to relaxation. It's hard to feel relaxed if you are lying on a terrible mattress or if you are stuffed to the gills, if you are worried about something or if you worked on your computer right up to bedtime.

We need to learn how to separate issues and events in our lives so each receives the attention it needs without detracting from the others. Learning to set aside other considerations when it's time to sleep is one of the most powerful things we can do for ourselves. The self-hypnosis discussion in chapter 7 contains a technique for deep relaxation. Use this if stress is one of the factors disturbing your sleep.

9. I've been told that I snore a lot, and loudly, too.

Snoring may get laughs on a TV sitcom, but it can be a real curse for those who must listen to it when they are trying to sleep. It may also signal a genuine problem that requires attention. If you are a regular and loud snorer, you may be suffering from a degree of apnea. Apnea means "without breath." This sleep disorder is discussed fully in the next chapter.

There are several reasons why someone might snore loudly. When we sleep, the muscles and surrounding tissues of our throat relax, and the air we breathe has to pass through a severely restricted passage. The air vibrates against the reduced opening of the throat, resulting in the classic raspy buzz we all have heard. Obstructed nasal passages can contribute to snoring, as can being overweight. Too much to drink before bedtime can do it, causing a deeper state of slackness in the muscle tissues than usual.

If you snore, try one of those nasal bandages you see sports players wearing, the kind that go across the bridge of the nose and hold open the nasal passages. This lets a lot more air in and reduces the amount of vibration. There is also a simple surgical procedure that can be performed in some cases to remove obstruction. See the section on apnea in chapter 3 for more information.

10. My legs get twitchy and jumpy when I'm asleep.

Some people suffer from a condition called Restless Leg Syndrome. With RLS, the person afflicted feels as if the skin is crawling or prickling on their leg or legs. The person moves their legs "restlessly" in an effort to make the feeling disappear. That in turn disrupts sleep. RLS is usually treated with drugs and may respond to herbal therapies. If you think you may have RLS, please see the chapters on sleep disorders and medications for more information.

11. I get enough exercise to feel good about myself and my health.

By now we have all been exposed to endless exhortations to exercise for our health. If you like to exercise, this isn't a problem for you, and as long as you don't overdo it, then your sleep is probably not affected. But if you are one of the many millions who find organized exercise distasteful, then this might be a factor in your sleeping patterns.

It's not necessary to try to turn yourself into Arnold Schwarzenegger. It's not even necessary to spend an hour or so working out on machines, treadmills, bikes, etc. All that is really needed is a regular, pleasant walk for a half-hour or so. Ideally, you should find time for a walk every day, allowing yourself to enjoy the scenery, whatever it may be, and not worrying about whether you are getting your heart rate up or increasing your metabolism.

Traditionally, Americans have not been great walkers, although Europeans have long understood the benefits of walking. Especially in our modern era of automobiles and other fast transportation, walking has become a lost art.

Regular, simple exercise is essential for a reasonably healthy body, and a healthy body is one of the key components of good sleep. You can choose any form of exercise that you think will benefit you, from a simple walk to a complex regimen. Whatever you choose, please make it enjoyable for yourself. Have fun with it and don't turn it into a contest with the part of you that just wants to relax. If you are not currently getting any exercise, then please consider it as another piece of the puzzle that will help you take charge of your sleep and well-being.

12. The temperature in my bedroom is just right.

The body likes different temperatures for different situations. Generally, cooler is better at night, providing it doesn't get cold. You should be able to adjust the temperature in your bedroom to suit whatever your preference is. This can get difficult, depending on the time of year. A hot, sleepless night is a classic experience for almost everyone.

I am not in favor of electric blankets during cold periods, although many people love them. A constant temperature is unnatural and is disruptive to sleep. Though the blanket is nice and warm and may help you fall asleep, you may wake up feeling unrested and groggy. If you have this problem, try getting rid of that blanket and go back to the old-fashioned, nonelectric variety.

Comfortable temperature is subjective, so your spouse or partner may like it a little hotter or cooler than you do. If that's the case, try to work it out so you both win. Fewer covers or more may do the trick. Layering blankets is probably a better idea than a "one size fits all" quilt, unless you both like the same temperature. That way you can adjust to changing temperatures according to personal preferences.

This may sound like a simple thing, but it's critical to comfortable sleep.

13. I like to work, read, and think things through in bed.

This one is tough to pin down. As with temperature, personal preferences make a lot of difference. Some people cannot sleep if they spend time in bed reading or watching television or working. Others feel that the bed is a comfortable "nest" where they can either relax with a book or get things done. Most sleep experts would recommend that the bed be left to making love and sleeping. Whatever your preference, if you are in a relationship, take into account your partner's preferences as well. They may be unwilling to tell you that your reading light is keeping them awake, or that they don't really relax until you are ready to sleep as well. In a relationship, communication about sleep preferences is just as important as it is with any other issue. It may be very important, because lack of sleep leads to irritability, anger, frustration, and other negative expressions that don't help people get along.

Working in bed is probably not a good idea, because you are programming yourself to think and act in a very linear, nonsleep manner. If you are someone who likes to work in bed, you may have noticed that when you lie down to sleep, it can be pretty difficult to turn off that part of the mind that is busy working and planning and thinking things through. Even when you finally fall asleep, there may be a kind of ongoing dream of work and worry that leaves you exhausted in the morning. If you're like this, see if you can break the habit.

14. I get sleepy during the day.

This statement is meant to draw your attention to the possibility that you may be sleep deprived without even knowing it. A majority of Americans are sleep deprived! We could also say a majority of Canadians, Russians, the British, the French, and so on. The odd thing is that many of us are unaware that we are not getting enough sleep.

Our cultural work ethic does not support sleeping well. Enormous work loads, long hours, swing shifts, "getting the job done," and deadlines act to keep sleep at bay. We all know napping on the job is a big no-no. The bad news is that the quality of our work has to suffer as a direct result of society's attitudes about sleeping and working. The best thing to be said about sleep deprivation is that it creates a subtle fog over our thinking and effort. At worst it can be deadly and dangerous, causing enormous mental, emotional, physical, and financial damage.

If you find yourself losing it an hour or so after lunch, try changing your diet. Avoid carbohydrates, like that loaf of French bread or that plate of pasta. Forget the big Mexican burritos and sopaipillas. Instead, go for high protein, light fare that will give you an energy boost and keep you alert during the rest of the workday. That chicken Caesar salad might be a good bet, but your typical fast-food burger and fries is a sure ticket to napville.

If you already eat lightly and with an eye to protein and energy, and you are still falling asleep, you are probably sleep deprived. Either you are not getting enough sleep, or the sleep you are getting is not refreshing or restorative. Follow the suggestions given throughout this book to improve your sleep, and you will be rewarded by a much different experience of work and play.

15. I have a medical condition that can wake me up at night.

There's not a lot I can say about this one, except that if you are one of the folks who fall into this category, you probably already know that this is a prime cause of interrupted sleep. Everyone will become ill from time to time, and this is usually disturbing to our sleep. Note that sleep is one of the instinctive and primal responses that the body produces when we are sick. Sleep restores and heals.

Temporary or chronic medical problems can certainly be a significant cause of sleeplessness. Self-hypnosis can be very effective in these kinds of situations. So can adjusting medication or using alternative techniques for relaxation and pain relief. Throughout this book are many suggestions and tips for helping you get to sleep. They apply equally whether you have a medical condition or not. Try out the ones that seem to resonate for you, and persevere. If one doesn't work, perhaps another one will.

16. I like to drink a lot of coffee during the day.

I like coffee. I used to drink a lot of it when I was younger, as much as a pot a day. If I tried that now, I wouldn't sleep at all! Coffee contains caffeine and caffeine is a stimulant. You already knew that, didn't you? So, what do you think happens when people drink coffee before they go to bed?

If you have ever traveled abroad, or if you are an evening person in a city where coffee and cafés are part of the nightlife, you know that many people are happily sipping espresso or cappuccino at a late hour. I guarantee you that they don't sleep well, though. There's a price to be paid for the enjoyment of that evening cup, and the price is restlessness until the caffeine wears off.

I used to drink espresso at night, but I also was on a work schedule that had me going home at four in the morning. The rule of thumb is to avoid coffee within about four hours before you go to bed. For me, that isn't long enough, as I am still stimulated (but tired!) even after four hours.

By all means, enjoy yourself with coffee, if that's what you like. Just be aware that it takes a while for your body to process the caffeine, and that you will not get much sleep until that process has been completed. If you've been drinking a lot of coffee and find it hard to go to sleep, changing just this one habit will bring rewarding results. It's your call.

17. I smoke, and I usually have a cigarette before bed.

I am not going to go into a tirade about smoking here. More than enough people are doing that, as you have probably noticed. If you don't smoke, then this isn't a problem in regards to your sleep. If you do smoke, please consider the fact that smoking is both addictive and a vaso-constrictor, and it will affect your sleep. A vaso-constrictor is a substance that closes down the circulatory system in some way. In other words, smoking restricts blood supply, especially to the brain. The brain is extremely sensitive to changes in blood flow, as it requires as much as ten times more oxygen than other parts of the body.

That last cigarette before bed feels good because it temporarily soothes the nicotine addiction. All smokers know this on an experiential level. Now you're relaxed, now you can sleep— except ten minutes later the brain is demanding more nicotine, and that begins to disturb the calming brain rhythms that precede and induce sleep. On top of that, the reduced blood flow makes the brain struggle to move through its normal processes of sleep and body regulation. This can lead to headaches, restlessness, wakefulness (moving around gets the blood moving more strongly), and more. Smoking is insidious in its effects. As an ex-smoker, I know.

If you smoke, try to cut back to a point where you no longer require that ten-minute hit and that last butt of the day. Of course, as all real smokers know, that is very difficult. You may want to consider going through the struggle of quitting. One of the benefits will be better sleep, once you get through the withdrawal period. During that withdrawal, sleep will be fitful, you will get cranky and tired—all "good reasons" to start smoking again. It's up to you. One thing is certain: you will sleep better if you quit.

18. My work schedule is regular and consistent, with the same hours every day.

If you work in a job where hours are regular and fixed, this isn't likely to be a cause of sleeplessness for you. But if you are one of the millions who works irregular hours or swing shifts, you can have a real problem with sleep. A common result of working swing shifts and changing schedules for work and sleep is insomnia.

The problem is that the demands of shift changes and irregular work/sleep hours confuse the circadian rhythms. For some, the solution may be to get another job, one with regular hours. But if that isn't an option for you, what can you do?

If you have to sleep during the day, all of the previous material about controlling your sleeping environment applies even more. Most important is darkness. A semi-dark room with the shades drawn against the sunlight isn't really good enough. You need a room that is *dark*. Do something to cover the windows thoroughly so light cannot enter.

Noises of the day are different from those of the night, and may include family and children, people entering and leaving the house or apartment, and outside noises like traffic. There is more noise during the day, so it's necessary to do something to block it out.

Establish and use a regular routine for sleeping during the day, as if you were going to bed at night. Do all the same things you would do at night and make sure you are as relaxed as possible before going to bed. Try to set up as normal a rhythm as you would have if you were working regular daytime hours. It can be difficult, so do your best. Anything that establishes routine and normalcy in your pattern of waking and sleeping will help.

I know an experienced pilot who works for one of the major airlines. His schedule is a nightmare of changes and stopovers, time differences and jet lag. He is a good example of someone with the worst possible combination of working hours, in terms of sleep. Needless to say (but I'll say it anyway!) he was having trouble sleeping. In fact he was lucky if he got three or four hours of sleep a night. I don't know about you, but I'm not terribly comfortable with the idea that the pilot of the airplane I'm on has been getting just a few hours of sleep a night. If you've ever seen the cockpit of a modern airliner, you can quickly imagine how easy it might be to flip the wrong switch or make the wrong decision if you were suffering from sleep deprivation.

The solution for the pilot was hypnosis. Combined with deep relaxation techniques that he could apply at home, hypnosis allowed him to regain a semblance of good sleep. He no longer suffers from insomnia.

The same can be true for you. Use chapter 7 to teach yourself techniques for relaxation and sleep.

19. I travel a lot in my work and often stay overnight.

Travel is usually very disturbing to our regular sleep patterns. It's okay if we are going off for a vacation in Tahiti—we can put up with the jet lag and odd sleeping needs for a few days while we mellow out on the beach. But most of us are simply dealing with the requirements of traveling for business and work. There isn't any decompression time on the beach to make up for the hassle.

I don't know of anyone who has been working for very long in a job that requires frequent travel who is happy about it. Travel gets old really fast when it's not for pleasure. Delays, hassles with flight schedules and departures, weather problems, airport trauma of one kind or another—and that's just the beginning! When the traveler arrives at the destination, who knows what joys await? If you're lucky you get a good, quiet room with a good bed and all the conveniences. But all too often, even at supposedly exclusive hotels, the experience is annoying and stressful.

If you've crossed several time zones, those circadian rhythms act up again. Plus, you probably had to get up early to make your flight, and you may have early meetings and a long, long day ahead of you. All of these factors are a setup for a bad night's sleep. Then, of course, you will have to adjust again when you return. The more this kind of traveling is a part of your life, the less likely it is that you will be able to sleep peacefully.

There are some things you can do; we talked about what you can do for jet lag in chapter 1. In addition, the key is to pay attention to your personal comfort and to follow a few simple rules when you arrive at your destination. For example, how many times have you lain down on a hotel bed and found that the pillow was a cross between a balloon and a cement block? You know the kind of pillow I mean: it's stuffed to capacity with foam of some kind and has the resiliency of a soft brick. Or, if it isn't like a brick, it's like a rubber sponge, bending and folding in every way except the one that is comfortable for you. A night on a pillow like this results in headaches, neck pain, and stress. You've got enough stress already. The solution is to take your *own* pillow with you, or something that works well for you to sleep on.

I can see all you hard-headed business people right now, saying, "Is this guy serious? Does he really want me to take my *pillow* with me? What would the guys in the office say about that? Do I need my teddy bear, too?"

What the guys in the office say doesn't matter. You will be producing great results in your work, thanks to the extra sleep you will be getting. And it will be because you had a decent pillow to sleep on while you were staying at that wonderful airport hotel your company booked you into.

One alternative to packing your pillow is to use a camping trick. Get a flannel pillow slip made for campers at your local outdoor recreation store. These are designed to be filled with something like a shirt or towel, and they work very well if you prefer a flatter kind of pillow than is normally found in hotels. You just put a couple of towels inside, and fluff it up to your satisfaction. This has the advantage of not taking up much packing room.

You can see from the above that I think pillows are critical for a good night's sleep. Along with things like not drinking alcohol or coffee near bedtime and doing whatever it takes to relax yourself after a day's travel, this is one of the best things I have ever found for helping me get to sleep at night on the road. It will work for you, too.

20. My mind is usually calm when I'm lying in bed getting ready to sleep.

This last one is a biggie, because many people can't stop think-ing about things easily when it's time to sleep. Remember what we said earlier about a "busy mind?" Being able to set aside the thoughts and concerns of the day at bedtime is one of the most important things you can learn to do to improve your sleep. If you already do this, great. If you don't, then this is a powerful change you can learn to make that will bring instant results.

If you answered **c** or **d** to this statement, you really owe it to yourself to break the pattern. There are a couple of ways to do that. First, take a look at your usual pattern before going to bed. Do you watch television until the last moment? If you do, avoid the "talking heads" shows and find something that is not very intellectually stimulating. That should be fairly easy. Do you have a bedtime ritual to help you make the transition from wak-ing day to resting night? By ritual, I mean a fairly routine and specific sequence of things that you do before bed. For most that means doing things like brushing their teeth, going to the bath-room, perhaps taking a shower—whatever it is, it should be a regular routine of some kind.

Routines of this sort may sound dull, but the mind likes rou-tines. Routines equal familiarity and security to the mind, and help it relax. Routines might not be a good idea when you are seeking change, adventure, challenge, or stimulation, but they are a great idea when you want to sleep.

If you do not have a routine, then create one. Do so with the conscious intention of preparing yourself for bed and for sleep. Don't just run upstairs, throw your clothes off, jump into bed, and expect to go to sleep quickly. It won't work.

If you have a particularly tough mind that wants to prepare for the next day and resolve all the outstanding issues of the pres-ent day, then you have to give it a chance to do its thing. By this I mean give your mind a way to satisfy the need for thinking through the problems and planning for whatever lies ahead. You can do that by creating a regular habit (ritual and routine again!) of sitting down and writing down what needs to be done and your comments on what has already happened. Make a list. Like routines, the mind loves lists. Lists don't help if you don't pay attention to them, but they can satisfy the mind's need to get organized and get attention for the things it feels are important.

You can make a brief list of what needs to be done tomorrow. Review the day and make comments to yourself about what happened. Write down any thoughts that will help integrate and settle the day's events. That way, when you lie down to sleep, you will not be carrying the day's baggage and tomorrow's plans with you in the same way. Try it, and you will probably find that it is much easier to drop off to sleep quickly, without having to worry about all of the details of your life. Self-hypnosis can help here as well. Please refer to chapter 7.

You can see from the sleep inventory that there are many ways in which you, personally, can take charge of the most important factors affecting your sleep. There is always some degree of personal intervention possible. This is true even when you have a medical condition or a physical problem that is affecting your sleep. You are the one who is in charge, always. You may not be able to change everything that might be affecting your sleep, but you can always find a way to modify it or adapt to it in ways that will produce better sleep and better results.

I think that the most important single factor in getting to sleep is a calm and relaxed mind. If you are worried about something, try your best to set it aside when it's time for bed. After all, worrying about it, whatever it is, is not going to change the situation, and it will be much easier to deal with the problem if you get enough sleep. Money, an emotional upset, work you have to accomplish—whatever the issue, lost sleep only makes it worse. Use one of the techniques given in these pages to calm your mind and open the door to healing sleep. You may find that the problem resolves itself easily in the light of morning.

CHAPTER THREE

SLEEP
DISORDERS

The best cure for insomnia is to get a lot of sleep.
—W. C. Fields

"Sleep disorder" is the name physicians and researchers give to a number of sleep disturbances. Most sleep disorders have a physiological or neurological basis, meaning that it may be necessary to consult with a physician to get relief. A few, like some kinds of insomnia and any disturbance that comes from a disruption in circadian rhythms (*e.g.*, jet lag), may be the result of psychological stress or external factors. Some, like apnea and sleepwalking, may be serious enough to be life threatening. What do these sleeping problems look like? How do you know when to see your doctor? What can you do about it if you have a sleep disorder?

Each sleep disorder looks a little different, and each has its own peculiarities and symptoms. If you recognize yourself in any of the descriptions that follow, you may want to consider seeing a physician about it. You can also get information and physician referrals from one of the centers scattered throughout the country specializing in sleep disorders. Consult the resources list at the back of the book to help find a center near you. Even if there is no center located near you, you may be able to call and get a referral to a physician in your area who understands the seriousness of your problem. Not all physicians are aware of the best treatments for their patients who are not sleeping well. Doctors tend to be overwhelmed with information and work, and they're only human—no one can be expected to know everything. You should find a doctor who is willing to do more than just prescribe a sleeping pill. You should always receive a full explanation of the nature of your sleep problem.

In the paragraphs that follow, you will find a description of just about every sleeping disorder that is commonly (and sometimes uncommonly) experienced by sleepless people everywhere. The list ranges from simple insomnia to life-threatening breathing problems. Since some symptoms overlap, a word of caution is needed: not all of these require medical treatment, so take the information with a grain of salt when applying it to yourself or someone you know. The important thing is to follow up on the information if you feel that you or a loved one has any kind of serious sleeping problem.

INSOMNIA

In pre-Christian times the Roman Empire eclipsed the Greek culture as the dominant force in the Mediterranean basin. With dominance came a whole new series of gods and goddesses, including a new god of sleep—Somnus. The Greeks' Hypnos was out and Somnus was in. From his name we derive our word for being unable to sleep, insomnia. Insomnia can make the sufferer completely miserable. Fortunately there are things that can be done to alleviate it. A few people suffer from life-long insomnia, but most of us are not so unlucky.

Insomnia is a broad term; for the sake of discussion, we can categorize many different "kinds" of insomnia. What they all have in common is loss of sleep. Depending on the particular symptoms that present themselves, a strategy or treatment can be devised to get things back to normal. Sometimes several of the different symptoms combine, making for a thoroughly miserable sleeping life.

Initial Insomnia

For many people just falling asleep easily is a big problem. If there are no interfering factors, most people will be asleep within seven to ten minutes after they lay down. Here's a good yardstick to measure by: if it takes you thirty minutes or more to fall asleep, you have initial insomnia. In chapter 2 several suggestions were given that can make a difference if you have trouble getting to sleep, such as adjusting or creating your personal sleep ritual, avoiding certain foods and beverages, and so on. Initial insomnia can be defeated relatively easily, if you can achieve a calm and relaxed state of mind before you get into bed. Pain or other physical problems must be dealt with as well. If you have chronic pain or other physical discomfort that keeps you awake, then I hope you are seeing a physician. More on this later, in the chapters on medication and self hypnosis.

Subjective Insomnia

Sometimes we have the feeling that we haven't slept at all, and wake up exhausted. This is called "subjective" insomnia, and it doesn't get a lot of respect from most sleep researchers. In the sleep labs the EEG and other instruments often indicate that subjects who complain of sleeplessness actually slept most of the night, in spite of the subjective report of not sleeping. The truth is that sleep scientists don't really know what to do with this. Their faith is in the "objective" readings produced by their machines, not the verbal reports of their subjects. I have never seen much intelligent discussion of this problem in research articles or books. At best, subjective sleeplessness is noted and dismissed as "anecdotal."

If you are someone who has subjective insomnia, it doesn't help much to be told that you really did get enough sleep after all. It's your experience that counts, not the objective description. There is always a reason for not sleeping well. In this case, try to eliminate any and all of the causes of poor sleep found in chapter 2.

Sleep Well, Sleep Deep

Chances are good this may do the trick. Smoking, alcohol, and high stress levels are all common contributors to the feeling of not having "slept a wink all night." Whatever the cause, know that you can almost always identify and eliminate it.

Psychological Stress-Induced Insomnia

Frequently, insomnia is caused by psychological stress. Some of the techniques talked about in the last chapter address the relief of stress. You can use them or the self-hypnosis techniques in chapter 7 to get relief.

Psychological stress can often be traced to a specific traumatic event. This kind of event can include anything in life that is disturbing or upsetting enough to really shake up our sense of personal safety and well-being. For example, anything that awakens our sense of personal mortality will create stress. There are many, many events in life that can do it, like an automobile accident, the death of a loved one, or a disturbing medical diagnosis. A brush with death or a severe injury, being the victim of a criminal act, witnessing something terrible, acts of nature (like tornadoes or hurricanes)—all these and more can stir up the psyche to the point where we find it difficult or impossible to sleep. Divorce or relationship problems, family illness, money difficulties, job worries—these, too, can keep us tossing and turning for hours as our mind gnaws away at the edges of the problem, trying to get to some kind of resolution.

There isn't any simple answer to getting past something like this. Some things, like grieving for the death of a loved one, have a natural timing and rhythm of their own that will not be hurried. Sometimes a problem resolves itself over time and sleep returns. Very often it helps to talk with someone about the particular focus of our concern. This might mean seeing a professional counselor for a while or perhaps joining a support group made up of others who have had similar experiences. Most cities and larger towns have various referral services and agencies that can provide help, if wanted. There are many free groups and service organizations that stand ready to help, because the people in them have been there, done that, and suffered through the same kind of stress. In the end sleep returns once we have come to terms with the event or resolved the problem, when we have been able to accept and integrate it into our lives.

Situational Insomnia

Another kind of insomnia is called situational insomnia. This occurs when we find ourselves in some unusual situation not in our control, causing anxiety and an inability to sleep. The key word here is control. A good example of something that causes situational insomnia is war. In wartime people lose the ability to directly influence events or predict accurately what will happen next. It's no surprise that people don't sleep well when they are being bombarded by missile or air attack, especially if warning times are short or nonexistent. The root cause of sleeplessness lies in the sense that one's personal safety is threatened and there is very little to be done about it. If the situation ends, sleep will usually return. It may take time for a normal pattern to re-emerge, especially if the situation is long-standing.

Most of us don't have to deal with living in a war zone, but we can find ourselves in dangerous and threatening situations just the same. Police officers, firemen, emergency response teams, people who live in dangerous areas, people who perform dangerous work—all of these and more are very likely to suffer from situation-induced sleeplessness. The best possible approach, barring a change in the situation (which may not be desirable or possible), is to learn techniques promoting relaxation and calm. Using these techniques regularly can alleviate the stress caused by the particular situation, and sleep will return.

Waking Too Early and Staying Awake

This is a common form of insomnia: you wake up at three or four in the morning, and then can't get back to sleep. Sometimes this is a side effect of the aging process. As we get older, we seem to sleep less and not as deeply. We don't spend as much time in deep sleep or REM sleep as we did when we were younger. Waking up early is also a common side effect of taking sleeping medications. If you are taking either over-the-counter or prescription sleeping medications, please read chapter 5 for more information. You will also find information there about melatonin and other nontraditional sleep aids. Melatonin, in particular, has been shown to be effective with older folks who are having trouble getting to sleep or going back to sleep when they wake up.

If you are someone who wakes up early, you may need to make a plan to adjust your sleeping habits or make changes in what you are doing. There are some key suggestions in chapter 8 that may be helpful to you.

Chronic Insomnia

Chronic insomnia is serious and debilitating. It can result from causes both physical and psychological. This can be very complex from a psychological standpoint. Just to give an example, have you ever known someone who has learned to manipulate others through their sleeplessness? We all sympathize and pay attention when people we know say that they haven't been sleeping well. It sounds crazy, but to the unconscious part of us that wants sympathy, it makes perfect sense to give up sleep in order to gain attention. If you know someone like this, you might consider gently suggesting that they seek professional help. You want them to feel that the idea is for them to recover their ability to sleep, not for you to feel less manipulated, so be careful!

A major cause of chronic insomnia is the use of sleeping pills. Sleeping pills are, at best, a way to break a cycle of sleeplessness and allow the normal rhythm to return. However, too often they are an addictive and inefficient stopgap measure. They should never be taken for more than a few days, but are often taken for weeks or months. After about two weeks, the body develops a tolerance for the drugs and the dosage may have to be increased, or a different medication prescribed. This creates real trouble when the pills are stopped or the dosage reduced. The body has come to depend on the drug to induce sleep (and it's not good, deep sleep at that) and now will not allow sleep without it. The result is insomnia. No pill will get to the underlying cause of the sleeplessness.

If you are regularly unable to sleep, you must determine the underlying cause before you can successfully break the pattern. Insomnia is a symptom, not a cause. Is the cause medical? Unless you already know that it is, you need to see your doctor to find out. Is it psychological stress? You may or may not know when you are experiencing a lot of stress. Amazingly, many of us haven't a clue that we have reached our limits. I often work with people who are simply unaware of how much stress really exists in their lives. They have concealed the knowledge from themselves, avoiding a confrontation with the underlying causes of their stress. For example, it may be difficult to make necessary changes that result in lowered stress and more sleep if the stress is a result of relationship problems or impossible work situations. It's easier to "stuff it" rather than face up to the situation and resolve it.

One way to find out if you are unconsciously stressed beyond your limit is to ask someone you trust if they think you are over the line. You may be surprised at the answer you get. Just don't bite the person's head off if he or she tells you that you seem "pretty uptight lately" or point out some other sign of high stress levels! Stress robs you of sleep, and sleep loss makes you feel stressed, so unless you break the cycle, it's going to be tough to get the sleep you need and deserve, much less relax and let go of the stress. Think about it, and then do something about it. Use any technique that works, aside from drugs or alcohol. Self-hypnosis, meditation, relaxation tapes, biofeedback, exercise—whatever it takes, it's worth the effort.

NIGHTMARES

I'm not going to say much about nightmares here, since the next chapter deals with dreams (and nightmares) in detail. Nightmares can be very disturbing to our sleep, as everyone knows. For now, consider the nightmare as (literally) a wake-up call to our outer awareness. Something is not right, and the nightmare is trying to get our attention. When we get the message, the nightmares will usually stop. More about this in chapter 4.

DELAYED SLEEP-PHASE SYNDROME

Delayed sleep-phase syndrome (DSPS) is what happens when our body clock gets reset to a later sleep cycle. It's easier to do than you might think. Perhaps you just can't resist those late-night get-togethers with your friends, or you get in the habit of staying up to watch the late show and then the late late show that follows it. Without knowing it, you are resetting your internal clock and training yourself to sleep at a later hour. If you decide to turn in early, you will then be unable to get to sleep. Unfortunately, you probably still have to get up and go to work the next day. This is one of the common effects of jet lag, and it's treated in pretty much the same way. You will have to make an effort to reset your clock back to its normal time. You can do that through light therapy or by readjusting your bedtimes and waking times until you are back on track.

When DSPS becomes chronic and disruptive to your lifestyle, serious attention is needed. The fix requires a conscious program of resetting your bedtime over a period of a week or so. This approach is called *chronotherapy*, meaning "time therapy." It sounds like something from *Star Trek*, but it works. For example, if you can't get to sleep before 4 A.M. and have to get up for work at 6:30, you've got a real problem. Sleeping pills won't do it. Chronotherapy might have you going to bed about three hours earlier each night for several nights, then going down to two hours earlier, then setting a regular time of 10:30 P.M. The adjustment takes place over a week or so. You can see that this approach requires dedication and a real desire to change the pattern.

DSPS is something you want to watch out for in children. It's easy for a child's internal clock to get set to an inconvenient hour, with resultant loss of sleep, crankiness, and so forth. That's not even counting the stress and struggle involved in getting the child to bed and to sleep. Don't let this pattern develop if you see it starting. More about children and sleep in chapter 6.

SLEEPWALKING

True sleepwalking in adults is rare and dangerous and requires serious attention. One of the most famous sleepwalkers of all time is Lady Macbeth. Shakespeare's manipulative and tormented character wanders at night, open-eyed and asleep, through the dreary castle halls, making washing motions with her hands. She tries to remove the blood of her crimes, blood she alone can see in her sleepwalking state.

The official name for sleepwalking is REM sleep disorder, because it is intimately associated with REM sleep. You will recall that REM stands for "rapid eye movement," and that this is the stage of sleep associated with dreams. We have four or five REM stages during any night, with an increasing duration of time in REM sleep as the night progresses. During REM sleep we are quite literally paralyzed, unable to move any of our major muscles. This is a good thing, because it prevents us from acting out our dreams. Imagine taking a swing at some dream attacker and finding out you have just punched your partner in the nose! If it were not for this protective paralysis, we could easily hurt ourselves or someone else. For the sleepwalker, however, this safety mechanism has somehow been turned off. The result is a danger of injury and even death.

It is not uncommon for children to sleepwalk. It's a phase that kids may pass through, and we deal with it by making sure they can't hurt themselves and by putting them back to bed. But in adults it can be deadly. Sleepwalkers have awakened to find themselves in very dangerous situations, and there are many reports of injuries. There are stories of people waking naked behind the wheel of their car, miles from home and with no idea of where they were or how they actually got there. People have climbed on the roof, walked into heavy traffic, stepped out of bedroom windows, acted out bizarre and frightening actions, attacked their would-be helpers or partners, and more, all while completely asleep and unconscious to the outer world. Even murder has taken place while sleepwalking.

Sleepwalking is something of a mystery. It does seem to be associated with a high degree of stress. Brain lesions may cause sleepwalking, or it may be the result of a malfunction in the brain stem; researchers are unsure why it happens. You can talk to someone who is sleepwalking, and they may or may not respond to you. You can try to verbally guide them back to bed, but you should not attempt to awaken a sleepwalker. It's best to stay out of their way—they can actually be dangerous to you. Try to ensure their safety by removing obstacles from their path or locking the door. Treatment is available, primarily with prescription muscle relaxants. One thing is certain: sleepwalking is a very serious problem and it *must* be treated by a physician.

NARCOLEPSY

Narcolepsy affects well over a quarter of a million people in the United States alone. Like sleepwalking, it's associated with the REM stage of sleep. In narcolepsy the sufferer immediately enters a REM state, rather than following the normal pattern where the REM stage occurs about an hour and a half after the onset of sleep. The person with narcolepsy is suddenly overwhelmed with an irresistible urge to sleep, or is constantly fighting off severe bouts of sleepiness. It doesn't matter how much sleep they get; the narcoleptic acts from time to time as if he or she never got any sleep at all. There can be sudden and frightening attacks of weakness and paralysis, called cataplexy (another good word for *Jeopardy* or a crossword puzzle). Even more embarrassing (if possible) is that these attacks can be brought on by emotions such as anger or any strong stimulus (like laughter), or even sex! You can imagine the scenario. There you are, all set for an enjoyable romp with your chosen partner when—*oops*, you fall asleep!

That's good material for a stand-up comedian, but it's not very humorous in real life. Narcoleptics have a terrible time holding down a job or functioning in most of the ways the rest of us take for granted. They can't do the things we do, like driving, swimming alone, or operating machinery. Sometimes attacks are accompanied by vivid and frightening hypnogogic hallucinations along with the paralysis. Narcolepsy seems to be gene-related and may indicate a brain stem dysfunction of some sort. It usually shows up in adolescence, and if it becomes an established pattern, it will always be present.

Treatment for narcolepsy is drug-oriented and two-pronged. The physician will seek to combat the excessive sleepiness with prescription stimulants and the cataplexy with other drugs. There have been good results in some cases with alternative approaches, specifically acupuncture and herbal remedies. As sleep scientists learn more, better techniques may emerge. This is another sleep disorder that absolutely requires the care of a physician.

APNEA

Apnea is a hidden killer, often overlooked and underdiagnosed. It's not necessarily the apnea itself that kills, but the effects of this disorder on the rest of the body, notably the heart and the circulatory and respiratory systems. Apnea means "without breath." Someone who has apnea literally stops breathing or has the breath blocked while they sleep. In severe cases, the sleeper can stop breathing hundreds of times during the night, and must "wake up" that many times to begin breathing again. You can imagine how it feels in the morning!

How do you know if someone has apnea? Have you ever seen a cartoon where the character is "sawing logs," perhaps with a word balloon overhead containing a word-sound like *ssnnkkxxx!?* Everyone knows this means snoring. A little snoring is okay and natural, but a lot of it means apnea. You may suspect that someone has apnea when he or she snores very loudly and consistently, every night. The person will also probably experience bouts of sleepiness during the day, even uncontrollably falling asleep at the worst times. Accidents have occurred when apnea sufferers fell asleep while driving. It is not uncommon.

There are three kinds of apnea, depending on how the symptoms appear. The most common kind occurs when the upper airway is blocked for some reason. Upper airway apnea is a straightforward blockage, not caused by the brain and not affecting the central nervous system. Treatment always involves reducing and eliminating the causes of the blockage.

The second and most dangerous type of apnea is called central apnea. In this form there is a complete halt in respiratory brain function. Breathing can sometimes stop for up to forty or fifty seconds, but usually for ten to twenty seconds. This causes carbon dioxide levels to rise in the bloodstream and oxygen levels to drop. When it reaches a certain point of saturation, the brain is triggered into waking the sleeper, which in turn starts the breathing process again. The third kind of apnea is really a combination of the first two; it may begin as a respiratory disruption but finish as an upper airway blockage. It is called, simply enough, mixed apnea.

Dr. William Dement thinks it's possible that SIDS, or sudden infant death syndrome, may be some variant of this adult sleep disorder. No one knows exactly what causes SIDS, but there appears to be a problem with the ability of the brain to regulate the vital functions. The adult wakes and stirs, restarting the breathing cycle, but the infant may not be able to do this. We are still deep in shadow when it comes to understanding how the brain functions in sleep.

Conservatively, there are at least twenty million people who suffer from apnea in the United States alone. There are serious personal side effects from apnea, aside from feeling tired and not getting restful sleep. One documented effect is a dramatic rise in blood pressure, along with an accelerated and irregular heart rate. Many people who have apnea are overweight and already suffer from hypertension. The additional stress placed on the heart by this sleep disorder is especially unwelcome for these folks, as it increases their already high risk of heart attack, stroke, and respiratory failure. The loss of oxygen to the brain caused by apnea can affect judgment and ultimately can even cause the loss of brain cells. This is especially bad news for children. If your child shows the symptoms of apnea, you must do something about it, or you run a very real risk of your child suffering brain damage and retardation, due to oxygen starvation.

The majority of people—by a factor of ten—who have severe apnea are overweight men. Losing weight is one of the fundamental treatments in many cases of upper airway apnea. It doesn't necessarily mean that large amounts of weight must be shed. Often just a few pounds can do it—it depends. Blockage of the airway (and the snoring that accompanies it) is usually a result of too much soft tissue (*i.e.*, fatty tissue) in the throat and the tongue. Sleep brings relaxation of the muscles that control the soft tissues. This allows the tissue to "collapse" into the airway, closing off breathing. The sound of snoring comes from the passage of air in and out through the reduced opening.

Excessive relaxation, such as when someone has had too much to drink, can produce snoring also, and for the same reason: the soft tissue collapses and the airway becomes narrow and obstructed. People who have upper airway apnea may struggle desperately for air, until the blockage is temporarily released, only to start up again as the tissue collapses back into the throat. This places a further strain on the heart and lungs and can shorten life span by a considerable amount.

Sometimes surgery is performed to remove the excess tissue and thus the obstruction. Currently, this is not much recommended, as it is limited in effectiveness. A few people have gotten excellent results from this, but for most the benefits are marginal. The earliest surgical treatments involved making a permanent opening in the windpipe—a tracheotomy. This works, but it is an extreme measure and is no longer used as a treatment of choice.

Today there is a very effective device that relieves the problem, invented by an Australian named Colin Sullivan. It's called a continuous positive air pressure machine (CPAP for short). The CPAP is a mask worn by the sleeper. The mask is attached to a machine that forces air into the nose, thus keeping the airway open. Sufferers from apnea swear by the CPAP. It finally allows them to sleep peacefully, something they may not have done in years. It only takes a few nights of good sleep to make a huge difference to our sense of well-being and happiness. CPAPs are becoming cheaper and more efficient, smaller and more available. If you have apnea, ask your doctor if one can be made available to you—while you do whatever else may be necessary to eliminate the problem.

Mild cases of apnea respond well to adjustments in lifestyle and eating or drinking habits. Mild weight loss, avoidance of alcohol or sedatives, and a regular routine for sleeping and relaxing will usually do the trick. In more severe cases, the CPAP and/or an aggressive weight loss program may be required. If you think you have apnea, talk with your doctor about it. If he or she is unresponsive, get a referral through one of the sources listed at the end of the book. You will be glad you did.

RESTLESS LEG SYNDROME

Sometimes called PLMS for "periodic leg movement during sleep," restless leg syndrome (RLS) is a very unpleasant sleep disorder that is almost always treated with drugs. When someone has RLS they have odd crawling or prickling sensations in their legs. It's as if insects were crawling on them! The response is to move the legs "restlessly" in an attempt to make the sensations go away. Of course it's hard to sleep when you are thrashing your legs about. It's also hard for your partner, if you are in the same bed.

As in so many sleep disorders, there is some debate as to the exact cause of RLS. Alcoholism and heredity may contribute. Other factors such as circulatory problems or diabetes may be present. In any case, it takes a physician to properly diagnose the treatment. RLS may respond to alternative therapies such as acupuncture or herbal treatment.

All of the sleep disorders described in this chapter have serious implications for our health and well-being. Each of them robs us of sleep, with all of the unpleasant consequences that follow. For many of these disorders, that is almost the least of the problem. As you can see, many require medical attention and are directly or indirectly life-threatening to ourselves or to those around us. If you suspect that you have any of the sleep problems listed above, please see your physician or talk to someone at one of the sleep-disorder centers listed later on. You owe it to yourself and your loved ones. Your life may quite literally depend upon it.

CHAPTER FOUR

SLEEP, DREAMS, AND HEALTH

THE FUNCTION OF DREAMS

T here is a lot of heated disagreement about the function and meaning of dreams. There are basically two camps: those who think dreams are significant and those who do not. Many scientists, sleep researchers, and even psychologists dismiss dreams as meaningless. If dreams are considered at all by the folks in this camp, they are usually seen as a reflection of random neurological "events," fallout from the brain's attempt to integrate and process the happenings of daily life.

My experience of working with dreams is markedly different. Twenty years of practical experience has convinced me that dreams have practical and useful meaning for our lives. I am quite sure that the "meaningless neurological event" description of dreams is scientific nonsense. I often discover critical information about the underlying problems that have brought clients to my office through the dreams they relate. Dreams are worth our careful attention.

There is a basic problem with the scientific approach when it comes to understanding the human psyche. It's in the nature of science to demand empirical, repeatable proof that something is so. Anything that cannot be nailed down in the lab, even if well documented and witnessed, will be considered "anecdotal." Anecdotal means just what it says: it's a story without hard proof to back it up, and therefore unacceptable for scientific consideration. Human awareness and consciousness, including dreams, does not lend itself well to empirical scientific understanding.

In general, I tell people that dreams are messages from ourselves to ourselves. We can trust the information the message contains, once we learn how to understand it. Since each person's life experience and history is unique, the symbols in our dreams most often cannot be interpreted in exactly the same way as they might be for someone else. This makes "dream dictionaries" and lists of dream symbols with "interpretations" practically useless. The skill in dream interpretation lies in understanding the personal meaning a dream symbol holds for the dreamer.

As an example, suppose that the ocean appears in a dream. What does it mean to the dreamer? To someone who has surfed and loved the water since childhood it means something quite different as a dream symbol than it does to someone who almost drowned in the ocean when they were five and has never returned since. The meaning of the symbol would be further modified by other factors in the dream, such as whether the ocean was calm or stormy, clear or muddied, shallow or deep, and so on.

Sleep research focuses on measurement and observation, with experimentation aimed at discovering the underlying biochemistry, neural mechanisms, and physiology involved. Dreams cannot be found in blood samples or EEG recordings. We may be close to understanding the physical processes of sleep, but it's another ball game when it comes to understanding dreams and their importance for our well-being.

Dreams occur during REM states of consciousness. One thing science has effectively shown is that REM sleep is critical for our health and sanity. A subject who is prevented from having normal REM periods of sleep, but is otherwise allowed to sleep normally, will begin to suffer very bizarre effects within a relatively short period of time.

If we don't get enough REM sleep, or if REM sleep is consistently disrupted, the first thing that goes is our ability to make clear judgments—just as if we were seriously sleep deprived. We become overwhelmed. Our memory suffers: we lose our ability to reason properly and think things through to a logical conclusion. After a few days of REM sleep denial, we start to hallucinate and act in very irrational ways. When finally allowed to sleep normally, we will immediately enter a long period of REM sleep and will be almost impossible to wake up. After a day or two, things will return to normal.

Is it dream deprivation that is creating these problems? No one knows. Dreams and REM sleep are inseparable, so there isn't a clear answer. Most scientific thinking focuses on the REM stage of sleep as a neural event and not on the dreams that accompany it. Researchers think REM states may be essential for storing and integrating memory functions and for processing daily information input to the brain. REM sleep is seen as part of an overall learning and brain maintenance process. Unfortunately, this process cannot be definitively understood. This leads to a lot of speculation, theoretical assumptions, and frustration from a scientific point of view. Since dreams are not a quantifiable aspect of sleeping and REM states, they are simply dismissed from consideration in favor of the neurological explanation.

To be fair to the scientists, traditional academic training and commonly accepted parameters of "credible" research prevent much serious thought being given to something as intangible as dreams. It's been left to others who seek to understand the secrets of the human psyche, rather than the mechanisms of the brain, to look more deeply at dreams. Dreams and sleep research may seem to be logical companions, but in fact they are worlds apart.

The other day I received an interesting request. It came from a doctor who was tired of not knowing what to say when his patients asked him about their dreams. I answered him with a short version of the ideas found in this chapter. What do you say to someone when they ask you what dreams are about or what their dreams mean? Do you know what your dreams mean? If you could understand your dreams you might be surprised at what you could discover about yourself. Along with issues of health, dreams will reflect any area of disturbance within the psyche, any part of our life where something is not working out as we would wish.

PHYSICAL HEALTH AND DREAMS

One of the most useful and practical things that dreams can do is signal physical illness. Over the years I have come across many dreams telling the dreamer something important about his or her personal health. I would go so far as to say that anytime we are threatened with a serious illness, our dreams will warn us that we are in danger.

The problem is that we often don't get the warning, because we don't understand the symbolic language of dreams. We have a built-in early warning system that alerts us to health problems in our dreams, but it doesn't come with a set of instructions. Just remembering dreams can be a problem, even without understanding their meaning.

Remembering dreams is fairly easy once we decide we want to do it. When we get the inner message across that we're interested, our mind will co-operate with remembered dreams. After that it takes practice and a little guidance to arrive at a genuine interpretation. Fortunately for us, if something is really important we are very likely to get a dream that is easily remembered, although we may not like it. This is one reason we have nightmares.

NIGHTMARES

Nightmares are a great way to get our attention. The word nightmare seems to come from the Middle Ages. People at that time thought such terrifying dreams were caused by evil spirits that literally rode on the back of the dreamer at night, like the back of a horse, thus the word "nightmare." We definitely remember our nightmares, because they are so shocking. We wake with the awful images planted firmly in our conscious mind. Dream images seem to be stored in very short-term memory locations in the brain. That is why we so quickly forget them. But a true, in-your-face, terrible nightmare will remain with us much longer than the average, garden-variety dream—perhaps permanently, if it is repeated more than once or if it is powerful enough.

There are lots of reasons why we might have a nightmare. All nightmares reflect some underlying disturbance in our being. Stress or difficulty in our lives, disease and illness (present or latent), disturbances in normal sleep patterns brought on by medication—all of these and more can initiate a nightmare. The important thing is to pay very close attention when we have one. The nightmare is literally a wake-up call to our outer mind, a message that something is wrong and we need to do something about it.

Nightmares are not caused by eating too much pizza before bed or by reading Stephen King. They are caused by fundamental psychological upsets within us that are independent of any immediate stimulus. Our mind may take images from the book (or even the pizza) and incorporate them into the dream, but it is not the book or the food that is the cause. Something may happen in our waking life that triggers the dream, but it is an underlying psychological dynamic that is reflected in the nightmare imagery. In the case of health dreams, the psychological becomes married to the physical: the nightmare tells us we are in trouble.

Life-threatening illnesses will appear symbolically in our dreams, usually some time before the outer symptoms appear or a diagnosis reveals the problem. Early diagnosis can make a big difference.

I have a friend trained in the scientific method (he is an M.D.) who has learned to pay attention to his dreams in a practical sense. You could say that he monitors his inner health and well-being through his dreams. He survived a bout with pancreatic cancer, normally a disease with about a 90 percent mortality rate. He knew something was wrong by the changing content of his dreams, which were nightmarish in quality. For him the undiagnosed cancer appeared as a series of disturbing tornadoes and threatening skies. The dreams prompted him to have the checkup that uncovered the disease.

A man with a life-threatening tumor in his head dreamed of a smoking television set; a woman I know with breast cancer has had dark and disturbing dreams both before and after the diagnosis. I have worked with many people whose dreams told them they were ill before they had actually been diagnosed. After the diagnosis, their dreams kept them informed about the progress of their treatment and the status of the illness. Mostly these have been folks with cancer, but other illnesses show up as well. Their dreams showed the inner disease process and then predicted the outcome.

The M.D. with pancreatic cancer had an extraordinary dream predicting the outcome of the very dangerous operation needed to save his life. He had not yet met the doctor who was to perform the operation. The night before the surgery, he dreamed that he was a passenger in his Jeep, driving across the wide ocean. A ruddy-complexioned man he did not know was driving. With some difficulty they drove across the great ocean together, reaching the shore. The next day he met his surgeon—and discovered that it was the man who had been sitting next to him in the dream! At that moment he knew he would survive.

In the case of the man with a brain tumor, a TV repairman showed up, indicating that the dreamer would get better. In fact, CAT scans that had initially revealed the massive tumor killing him later showed complete remission. The breast cancer patient has had dreams that indicate a potential for healing, symbolically portrayed as flowers blooming in the desert. For the moment, she has been diagnosed as being cancer-free.

Part of the difficulty in understanding dreams and nightmares is that symbols seen in dreams cannot be interpreted with a consistent meaning that applies to everyone. Not all dreams of tornadoes or televisions mean the dreamer has cancer! Each of us has his or her own symbolic dream language, composed of images that have particular meaning for us. One person's meaningful symbol may not be very important for another. It takes practice and guidance to become good at understanding your dreams and the dreams of others.

You may remember that I said earlier we have a built-in early warning system to alert us to health problems in our dreams, but that it doesn't come with a set of instructions. Here's a set that might work for you, if you are interested. By following the instructions, you may be able to discover something about yourself and your health. It's possible to monitor the true state of your health this way, but don't forget the part about regular physical checkups as well! Dream interpretation is not a good substitute for professional evaluation and diagnosis. On the other hand, it can lead you to early discovery of a potential problem, so it's worth the trouble to learn something about it. It does take practice, so have fun with it.

DREAM INSTRUCTIONS

1. Prepare yourself to record your dreams.

First of all, get ready to record a dream when you have it. Keep a pad and pen near the bed. When you wake with a dream, write it down. Keep a small flashlight also, so you don't have to turn on the light to see what you are writing. Night writing in the dark can result in some very interesting and illegible scrawls by daylight. My favorite way of capturing dreams is to have a small tape recorder ready. Then I don't need a light at all, as long as I make sure to turn on the record button. If you use this technique you will be amazed when you listen in the morning at what you have forgotten. After listening, write the dream down. Waking up briefly to record the dream will not disrupt your sleep, as long as you don't turn on the light and get involved in writing it all down. That is one reason I prefer a tape recorder to a writing pad.

Keep a dream journal. This is simply a notebook where you record all of the dreams you remember and your thoughts about them. Over a period of time certain scenes or images may reappear. By looking at these you can begin to get a sense of the underlying themes of the dreams, especially if they involve health issues. If an image or series of images appears again and again, pay attention. If an entire dream repeats, pay attention. Sometimes a dream repeats a theme, but not in exactly the same images. The similarity shows up when you review what you've written. If that happens, treat it as a recurring dream and pay attention. Recurring dreams are emphasizing a particular message or piece of information important for you to know and are seriously trying to get your outer mind to act accordingly.

2. Prepare yourself to remember your dreams.

It doesn't help a lot to have recording materials ready if you don't remember what you dreamed. This may not be a problem for you—some people find it easy to remember—but most of us forget and recall little or nothing. Dreams are stored in very short-term memory and may literally be forgotten in seconds. Making a conscious effort to remember alerts your mind to the idea that you actually are interested in what your dreams have to say. You can learn to remember many dreams on any given night. Each REM period of sleep is accompanied by dreams, and we have four, five, or more REM periods each night. As the night progresses, the period of REM sleep lengthens. Many of the dreams we easily remember occur during the last period before we awaken in the morning.

Try this to help you remember: as you down to sleep, give yourself a simple suggestion. Say to yourself, "Tonight I will remember my dreams." Repeat this several times, and at the

96

same time press your hands gently onto the center of your chest. Each time you repeat the phrase, "Tonight I will remember my dreams," press your hands onto your chest. This helps to "anchor" the suggestion by adding the feeling of physical touch. Do this every time you go to bed, as you are drifting off to sleep.

This is a simple and very effective technique. Most people report success in remembering dreams and dream fragments within a few days. Sometimes it happens right away; sometimes it takes a couple of weeks. Be patient and make sure you have your recording materials handy. You will eventually be rewarded with a dream. When you have it, no matter how insignificant or short it may be, write it down in as much detail as you remember.

Details are important. The color, the sound, the setting, the light—anything and everything is meaningful, especially when you are learning how to make dreams a useful part of your life. Record it all, including any feelings, emotions, or thoughts you may have had during the dream.

3. Think about the images in the dream, and let your mind free-associate with them.

"Free association" means to simply allow thoughts or feelings to surface that are "associated" with the dream image. It was Sigmund Freud who reinitiated this technique in modern times. It has always been the basis of good dream interpretation. Interpretations have always been couched (with apologies to Dr. Freud) in the cultural imagery of the time and place of the dreamer. The particular belief systems and theories of the interpreter will color an interpretation.

Ancient Greeks thought the gods were speaking to them, but Freudians think in terms of the primal and irrepressible urges of our instinctual selves. Jungians see dreams in terms of archetypal images and a collective unconscious; modernists tell us we can and should control our dreaming life consciously and enjoy the ride. Your interpretations will be based on the images, values, and cultural context in which you live. The trick to successful inter-pretation is to get past the surface associations to the underlying psychological meaning. Only practice can develop this skill.

For example, suppose you have a dream of finding yourself naked in public. This is a very common theme in dreams. All of us are very much the same under the skin, and there are some dream events that tend to show up for almost everyone—this is one of them. Free association allows you to think about what this image means. You are naked, you are embarrassed (or not—it depends on the dream), you feel like hiding or you step into public view, you feel exposed, exposure means that something is revealed, you are or are not concerned about it, and so on. Depending on the way in which you acted and felt in the dream, you could come up with a couple of possible interpretations based on your associations with the images.

If you are embarrassed and want to hide, then perhaps you fear "being exposed," *i.e.*, being found out, or being seen as inadequate or feeling unprepared for something that will be seen by the "public." The public can be a symbol for anyone who is not you and who may see you in some way; the public could also be referring to an inner sense of self-criticism or evaluation. There will always be some association in a practical sense with your waking, outer life. Perhaps you are faced with a big pres-entation at work, or are unprepared for an upcoming test of some kind. This stress shows up in the dream images. If you are comfortable in the dream and unconcerned, perhaps you are feeling secure about yourself, unafraid of being seen, etc. See how it works?

4. Make an initial interpretation.

This is an extension of step number three above. After you associate dream feelings and images with ideas and feelings about yourself and your outer life, you come up with a conclu-sion, a reading of the message of the dream. In the example above, you might realize that you were feeling quite out of your depth regarding some external event, like a work presentation or a test you are worried about. Once you arrive at the message, you have practical information you can work with. In this case, it might mean taking steps to reduce stress levels or reviewing the work you have done to be sure you're prepared. It could mean that you just acknowledge the stress and move on. It's up to you, but the dream will have told you something truthful about your inner mental state.

Dreams symbolically present the inner truth about how we think and feel, along with timely and accurate reports on our physical well-being. Good health may be reflected in dreams of joyful events and pleasant adventures. When health deteriorates, it's a different story. It's a little harder to identify health dreams.

5. Decide if the dream is about your health.

Our dream instructions get a little fuzzy here. Health dreams can range from the simple to the complex. They are not necessarily easy to spot or understand. When you are first starting out with dreams, it's important to take your ideas about them with several grains of salt. Keep a sense of humor, and pay as much attention to the feeling of the dream as to the logical interpretation.

Using this as a broad rule of thumb, it makes sense to pay more attention to dreams that upset or disturb us. Such a dream may be the first sign we get that something is going wrong in our physical body. It can be a nightmare that gets our attention. It can also be a dream that leaves us uncomfortable without knowing why. The woman I mentioned earlier with breast cancer had several vague and disturbing dreams, dark in nature without being fully remembered. She felt threatened and uneasy. These dreams foreshadowed the actual diagnosis by some months.

Not every dream that upsets us is addressing a direct disease process like cancer, but every dream that upsets us does address something internally that can lead to specific health issues. An example is high stress. Stress will show up in our dreams, perhaps as a nightmare. In itself, high stress is not considered a disease, but it can lead to illnesses like hypertension, stroke, heart disease, and asthma.

How can you tell if a dream is referring to your health? There isn't a hard and fast answer, but there are some general guidelines you can consider. As with all dreams, you have to be careful what meaning you give to the dream images. Some images I have seen over the years tend to repeat themselves with different dreamers and may indicate health problems. A word of caution here—if any of these images are appearing in your dreams, it does *not* necessarily mean that you are ill or have a disease! Remember, dream symbols can mean many things. A dream of sharks attacking could symbolize a disease or it could mean that the dreamer is feeling threatened by business competitors—or something completely different. A dream of a tornado approaching could easily symbolize an inner emotional storm or disturbance and have nothing to do with our physical health.

Devouring animals often appear in health dreams, especially primitive forms. Sharks, strange fish with teeth, snakes, crabs, alligators, scorpions and spiders, nameless things that menace and slither and attack the dreamer—these are common. They will almost always be accompanied by a feeling of menace and fear. The inner self knows when it is in danger of physical extinction and will make it clear in the dream world.

Once in a while a figure may appear in our dreams and direct our attention to something that symbolically represents a disease or a health problem. Foods and habits that are bad for us might be singled out, like eating too much sugar (not good if you are potentially diabetic, for example), smoking, drinking too much alcohol, or taking drugs. If you get such a dream figure, take notice, because this is one of the easiest health-oriented dream themes to spot. Such figures may appear to teach us other things as well, but try to get a feeling for what the image means when you are reviewing the dream. You can often get a good sense of the hidden meaning and what it's about.

There are times when we may hear a voice, as if off-stage, telling us to pay attention to something. There does seem to be some aspect within us that can appear in dreams and give us direct and good advice. If you see such a figure in a dream, try to record everything about it and to remember the message. These are important dreams to think about.

Symbols representing our body or different organs will appear in our dreams if needed. In the example of the man with the brain tumor, the television set was a very good symbol to represent his brain. Think about it: a televison receives and displays information and acts as a vehicle for communication. It makes a good metaphor for the physical brain and all of its functions. It could just as well have been a computer, for the same reasons. Because the set is smoking and sparking in the dream, we know that there is a serious problem. Because the repairman shows up, we know there's a potential for healing. The key to understanding the dream is to correctly interpret the symbol of the television.

Dreams of suffocating, being crushed, or drowning may be associated with heart and lung diseases, although they could also refer to a "suffocating" or "crushing" situation in the dreamer's life. If you have such a dream, take an honest personal inventory of yourself and your physical condition. Are you out of shape? Do you get short of breath very easily? Are you tired all the time? Do your feet and hands get cold a lot? Is your sleep erratic and disturbed? Coupled with a warning dream, these would be very good indications that it's time to set up an appointment with your physician, just in case you are developing heart, circulatory, or other problems.

Sometimes dream images will appear of dark, dirty, and trashed-out neighborhoods, houses, and streets. Houses are wonderful symbols for many different aspects of our lives, including the physical body. Dream houses can be old and abandoned, neglected, full of garbage and debris. When cancer has spread through the body, this is an image that can appear. But let me remind you—just because you dream of a neglected house, it does not necessarily mean you have a health problem.

If you have been diagnosed with an illness, your dreams can keep you posted on the success or failure of treatment. By observing the way the dreams progress, you can see if it's working or not. For example, is the garbage being cleaned up? Does there appear to be a new look, a brighter look to the buildings? This is when interpretation gets murky, because cleaning up the debris could also signal preparation for death, getting ready to go. The dreams have to be kept in perspective, taking into account all of the other factors that are present.

When someone is terminally ill, they will very likely have a dream of completion signaling when the end is at hand. Sometimes medications prevent this from happening or being remembered. Such dreams often reveal hope for renewed life in a spiritual realm. If we are getting ready to let go of a loved one, such a dream can help prepare us (and the patient) for the transition.

Recently, I saw a televison program that included dreams about dying and life after death—perhaps you saw it also. One dream in particular stood out for me. An elderly, dying woman dreamed that she saw a lit candle in her room, on the inside of her window, which was closed in the dream. The candle flickered and died out, only to reappear a moment later, relit—but on the other side of the window. This is a classic death dream, at the same time holding out the idea of renewal and spiritual rebirth. A truly wonderful dream, consoling and easing the woman and, in fact, signaling her death. She woke and told the attendant of her dream, then died very shortly after.

DREAMS, PSYCHOLOGY, AND ILLNESS

Health dreams often present an internal, psychological solution that is required to support the healing process. This is a gray area in medicine, because there is dispute about the role psychology may play in illness. For myself, I am completely convinced that the two are inseparable. More and more doctors are realizing that our personal psychology and our perceptions about who we are and our role in life have something to do with the illnesses that we contract and with the progression or remission of disease. Some doctors would say that there is a direct cause-and-effect relationship between how we feel about ourselves and our physical health, but most would not go that far. Whatever the truth may be, my experience is that when we are ill our dreams may present us with both the underlying psychological causes of our illness and with potential solutions that can lead to recovery.

I have worked with the dreams of several women who had breast cancer. Anyone who isn't living in a cave knows that breast cancer is a major killer and a brutal blow to a woman's sense of self. The diagnosis is fearful, the prospects disturbing in spite of the bright optimism seen in TV commercials promoting regular examinations and mammograms. Once diagnosed, treatment ranges from the invasive to the destructive, with all of the standard cancer tag alongs of radiation, chemotherapy, drugs, and surgery.

All of these women had dreams that indicated the presence of the cancer. All of them also had dreams that seemed unrelated to the illness from a causal point of view, but which actually pointed out the root psychological causes contributing to the development of the disease. I can't prove it, because dreams and their interpretations don't fall into the same category as cancer cells under a microscope do, at least not in a sense that medical science can accept. Let's just say that dreams reflect an inner reality that is a mirror of outer reality. A healthy body has healthy dreams, but a body racked with illness does not. Dreams may reveal both the reality of disease and the possibility of remission, if remission is an option for that person.

Whether or not there is an option for physical remission revealed in dreams, there is always an option for a return to a personal sense of harmony and reconnection to life and spirit, even if death is inevitable. Dreams will point the way and prepare us for the transition from life, if that is what must be. Traditional cultures throughout the world honor this aspect of dreaming and healing. In many Native American traditions, for example, healing does not necessarily mean physical recovery. It does mean a return to a sense of right connection with all living things, with family, clan, and nation.

If you have been diagnosed with a physical problem, you can help yourself through it by paying attention to your dreams. Try out the simple steps outlined above and make an effort to let the feelings about the dream come to the surface. It's possible to read meanings into dreams that aren't really there, so be gentle with yourself and simply take time to consider what your dreams may be trying to tell you. With practice and good intention you can get valuable and practical information that may help you get well.

This completes our brief set of dream instructions. As you can see, it's an interesting and often difficult task to determine the true meaning of a dream. If you find yourself getting a series of powerful dreams that stick in your waking mind, see if you can find someone to help you understand them. Be wary of pat interpretations and try to get to the feeling behind the dream. If it's important enough and if you have good intentions, you will eventually discover the truth. It's worth the effort.

HYPNOGOGIC STATES AND DREAM PARALYSIS

A hypnogogic state can occur as we are slipping into Stage 1 sleep or emerging from sleep. In the last chapter I talked about REM sleep disorder and how there is a mechanism in the brain that serves to paralyze muscle functions during REM sleep. If we did not have such a mechanism, we would act out the motions in our dreams and injure others and ourselves. That is what happens during REM sleep disorder.

In a hypnogogic state we are actually paralyzed, because the mechanism that shuts off major motor functions is operating to protect us from acting out our dream. We find ourselves in what is in effect a waking nightmare. We believe ourselves to be awake (although we are not) and at the same time are experiencing visual, auditory, and tactile hallucinations. We don't know that these are hallucinations. We may think people are in our room talking, or we may see things. All the time we are unable to move, yet we believe we are wide-awake and not asleep. This is an absolutely terrifying experience.

People tend to enter hypnogogic states when they are under severe stress. It's a warning sign that we've gone too far, that we need to lighten up and break free from whatever it is that has us so stressed out. It takes a lot of stress, not just a little, to bring on this state.

If you have had this experience, you know how awful it is. Most people think they are in danger of going crazy, because the hallucinations are so real and the feeling of paralysis so devastating. If this happens to you, it's a signal to do something about your life, right away. Don't treat it as an option, but take the steps, whatever they are, to change things in your life so that the stress levels subside.

POST-TRAUMATIC STRESS DISORDER AND DREAMS

Post-traumatic stress disorder (PTSD) is a real psychological ailment now becoming more frequently diagnosed. It is almost the psychological disorder *du jour* in our frenzied and stressed-out society. The symptoms include erratic and disturbed sleep, nightmares, depression, inability to function effectively in the world, irrational fears, and more. A goodly number of war veterans suffer from PTSD, as do many other people who have gone through some traumatic and life-threatening experience. It isn't necessary for the person to actually have been physically in danger: it's the perception of personal vulnerability and personal helplessness that underlies the symptoms. For example, in the aftermath of the Oklahoma City bombing many people not directly involved have been diagnosed with PTSD.

Dreams accompanying PTSD are often nightmarish and disturbing, frequently including repetitive dreams. Dreams repeat when there is a particularly important theme that the unconscious mind wants to get across to our waking self. It seems that something inside us wants the message to get heard and acted upon, and until that happens the dream will recur as needed. In PTSD, dreams present a picture to the dreamer of the underlying fear and stress forming the heart of the disorder.

I remember one client who came to me with PTSD and a terrible dream that had kept him awake for over twenty years. I'll call him Bob, although that was not his real name. Bob was a Vietnam vet, one of the thousands of young men who found themselves in the miserable hell of that misguided war. A combat Marine, he was just nineteen years old when he found himself in the midst of the Vietnam jungle, surrounded by a dedicated enemy that wanted to kill him.

Bob was at the end of his rope. Every time he went to sleep he would have the same nightmare. He found himself back in Vietnam, on patrol. The dream was intensely realistic, and as it progressed the sense of danger and fear would increase. The dream almost exactly replayed an actual incident from the war. In real life a sudden artillery attack literally blew up the man next to Bob, drenching him in blood, ruptured organs, and torn bits of flesh. In the dream the same event was repeated again, playing itself out until Bob would awaken screaming and drenched in sweat, sometimes striking out at his wife beside him.

I don't know how he managed to survive twenty years of this. He had the dream *every* time he went to sleep. This meant that every night he would wake up after about an hour or an hour and a half of sleep. He had not slept for a longer period at a single stretch in all that time. Most of us would have quietly retired to the looney bin long before Bob found his way to me.

What emerged in our conversation was the story of what had happened to Bob in Vietnam. It wasn't the first time he had told the story. The dream was obviously trying to get something across to him, but what was it? Was he just "having a nightmare" about Vietnam, as so many vets do? Nothing had worked for him over the years to bring about any kind of resolution.

Bob's psyche had somehow gotten "stuck" at the moment of the explosion next to him and was repeating the scene over and over in the dream, like a dog neurotically chewing on a bone. Why?

The answer, as it turned out, was deceptively simple. Remember that Bob was only nineteen years old at the time he was covered in blood. One moment his buddy was standing there, the next he was blown to bits. It was random and instant. It was out of control. *It could have been Bob.* In that moment Bob's sense of immunity vanished, and he knew he was mortal. It's not that he thought about it in that way, but something inside him knew it was true and it "freaked." Right there is where he got stuck.

Mostly nineteen-year-olds do not think in terms of mortality, even combat soldiers carrying the power of life and death in their hands. Teenagers tend to feel immortal, because they don't really believe death and personal extinction can happen to them.

That moment of the explosion was a moment of truth for Bob's immature and adolescent self, and it couldn't handle the reality. In an effort to understand and integrate the experience, it gave him his dream. He had never consciously realized before that this instant in Vietnam was actually a major turning point in his perception of self and his personal relationship with life. Before that moment, he was safe; after it, he never felt safe again. When the recognition dawned on him during our session, he cried deeply. He went home and slept for eight hours straight, for the first time in twenty years. The dream never returned, although he still sometimes had disturbing nights.

If you have a disturbing and repetitive dream, and if you have been diagnosed with PTSD, there is a key to your personal healing contained within your dream. Try to find someone who knows how to work with dreams to help you understand the meaning. There aren't too many trained people practicing dream interpretation, outside of some psychoanalysts. Psychoanalysis is not for everyone and requires a long-term commitment. If that's not for you, see if you can get a recommendation from someone who has had good results working with their dreams and has found a guide for the journey. It can pay off in better health and increased self-understanding. After all, what have you got to lose?

LUCID DREAMING

Lucid dreaming, or conscious dreaming as it is sometimes called, is perhaps the one area of dreaming that is subject to serious research and accepted as such by sleep researchers. The main work being done with lucid dreaming takes place at Stanford University, at the same sleep labs headed by Dr. Dement. The best known figure in lucid dreaming research is Dr. Stephen LaBerge, founder of the Lucidity Institute.

Lucid dreaming happens when the dreamer learns to awaken within a dream, realizing consciously that he or she is still dreaming. At this point of consciousness or lucidity, the dreamer can make choices about how the dream will progress. An entirely new dream can be created, potentially any dream possibility the dreamer desires.

Proponents of lucid dreaming advocate using the technique to address all sorts of psychological issues like nightmares or stress. Rather than attempt to understand the meaning of a nightmare, a lucid dreamer might choose to confront and conquer the nightmarish fears or change the dream so that threatening monsters become harmless friends. This technique has been practiced for centuries by a native tribe called the Sennoi. Theoretically, lucid dreaming can also be used to speed cellular healing or to attack cancer cells. It's all the same in principle— the dreamer decides what it is he or she wants to accomplish and sets out in the dream to do it.

Lucid dreamers train themselves to respond to certain cues in a dream that trigger the lucid condition. One way to do this is to develop a visual cue while awake that later appears in a dream, acting as a signal to the dreamer to shift into lucidity. Sometimes a light device may be used to trigger entry into the lucid state or to signal researchers that such a state has been entered. Interesting, since the subject is asleep! You can see why people might be attracted to the technique. If you could have any dream you wanted, what would it be?

I personally am not an avid supporter of lucid dreaming, since I find so much benefit in allowing dreams to take their natural course and reveal the workings of the inner self. It's a personal choice. If you are interested in lucid dreaming you can find more information about it in the library or bookstore. There are also many sites on the Internet that address the subject.

To close out this chapter, I'd like to leave you with one thought: dreams are meaningful and important. If you are a person who has vivid and frequent dreams, you have direct access to an amazing resource of wisdom and personal understanding. If you are ill, your dreams will reveal the truths of your illness, as well as the underlying psychological dynamics that might be involved. If you are healthy, your dreams can help you solve problems of life and relationship. If you are having trouble sleeping, any dreams you have may well reveal the causes of your sleeplessness. Honor your dreams, and you will be rewarded with understanding.

CHAPTER FIVE

SLEEPING PILLS, HERBS, AND OTHER SLEEP AIDS

MODERN SHAMANS

Sleeping potions have been around for a long time. In the ancient world the gift of sleep was one of the few medications that healers of the period could count on. Many effective preparations were made with opium extracted from the Eastern poppy, but other herbs and flowers were widely used as well. From the Amazon jungle to the steppes of Mongolia, from the plains of the American West to the mountains of Africa, native cultures discovered and used plants to bring on healing sleep. In those earlier times every culture had its shamans or medicine healers who knew the secrets of nature's gifts.

Some of those traditions still survive, but today most of us no longer live in a society closely attuned to nature. We do not understand the benefits and dangers of herbal remedies. If we can't sleep we don't consult our local shaman. We are far more likely to pick up a nonprescription sleeping aid at the local grocery store, carelessly tossing some brightly colored box touting peaceful sleep into our cart with the eggs and diapers.

If we are really having trouble sleeping we might ask our doctor to prescribe something stronger. Unlike the shaman, a modern physician relies on the synthetic products of the pharmaceutical industry to do the job. But when are sleeping medications the best way to deal with sleeplessness?

A good medical practitioner will not immediately reach for the prescription tablet if a patient has trouble sleeping. Because there are so many possible reasons for sleeplessness, common sense demands that the doctor probe for possible medical, lifestyle, or psychological causes that might be contributing to the problem. If the reason you can't sleep is because the neighbors upstairs are playing their stereo at two in the morning and keeping you awake, a sleeping pill is not the right treatment.

Different kinds of sleeping problems require different medications and different approaches, if medication is called for. If the patient has one of the neurologically or physiologically based sleeping disorders described earlier, that will determine what may be prescribed. The importance of accurate discussion and diagnosis of the root cause of the sleeping problem is critical. You can help your doctor and yourself by being fully prepared with the key information your physician will need to know. Here's a brief checklist of things to think about and questions to ask yourself before you go in for your appointment.

Getting Ready to Speak With Your Doctor

—— Make a list of specific symptoms and things you have observed about your sleeping habits. What does the problem "look" like? Describe the feeling and the circumstances. For example, perhaps you wake up many times during the night and feel dull and listless in the morning. What have you done to try to deal with it so far?

—— Are you tired during the day? If so, is it all day long or only during specific times?

Sleeping Pills, Herbs, and Other Sleep Aids

—— If you do not sleep alone ask your sleeping partner if he or she has noticed anything out of the ordinary. For example, do you snore loudly and often? Are you suddenly sitting up in bed at night gasping for breath?

—— Do you have nightmares or night sweats? If so, for how long?

—— Are you currently taking any over-the-counter medications or other remedies to help you sleep?

—— Are you under a lot of stress for some reason?

—— Chronic physical problems, such as asthma or hypertension, may make it difficult to sleep. If you have one of these problems, are you taking any medications for it?

—— Are you taking any other prescription medications?

Be prepared to briefly and accurately discuss anything revealed by the checklist above. Most doctors will pay close attention if a patient complains about loss of sleep, because sleeplessness can mask many possible problems. If for some reason your doctor doesn't seem to respond as you would like, insist on a recommendation. If you are not happy with the advice, seek another opinion. Make sure your physician understands how important it is for you to get the sleep you need. Many of the sleep disorders described in chapter 3 require a specialist for effective treatment. You can refer to the resource section at the end of the book for some help in finding a sleep-disorder specialist if needed.

Once external causes of poor sleep like noisy neighbors, too much coffee, or bad mattresses have been eliminated as a cause, the search for sleep solutions turns in other directions. Medical problems require treatment. Psychological problems like stress or depression that affect sleep may also need to be addressed.

113

Sometimes medications given to alleviate a physical or psychological problem can interfere with normal sleep. For example, some drugs affect secretion and reuptake of the hormone serotonin, a neurotransmitter responsible for many different tasks, including initiating the onset of sleep. The release of serotonin is in turn triggered by the production of melatonin and other substances like tryptophan (more about melatonin and tryptophan later in this chapter). The only way to know if the medications you are taking might interfere with your sleep is to ask your physician or pharmacist. Don't hesitate to ask, and don't assume that your doctor already knows what you're taking, or what side effects there might be regarding your sleep.

PRESCRIPTION SLEEPING MEDICATIONS

Over the years there has been a continuing evolution in the kinds of sleeping medications prescribed. There are several different types of prescription sleeping meds. Each has varying effects and its own particular set of necessary cautions. All of them are potentially dangerous if used over long periods of time; for many formulas a "long period" is anything more than two weeks. Almost all prescription sleeping aids have a severe effect on REM sleep and can prevent or disrupt Stage 4 deep sleep. In many cases physical addiction is a very real danger and can occur quite rapidly as the body builds a higher and higher tolerance for the drug. Beyond physical addiction there is also the danger of psychological dependency. Like cigarettes or booze, even if the physical addiction is broken, a strong psychological craving can remain.

The most dangerous class of sleeping drugs is the barbiturates. Once very common, they are now not as frequently prescribed. These drugs, with brand names like Nembutal and Seconal, are highly addictive and can have serious side effects when withdrawn. Today most sleeping prescriptions are in a class called benzodiazepines. These are considered "hypnotics" and act by depressing the central nervous system.

114

Sleeping Pills, Herbs, and Other Sleep Aids

Benzodiazepines are also used as sedatives and tranquilizers. This class of drugs can further be broken down into two kinds: those that are considered short-acting, or with a short "half-life," and those with a long-acting or long half-life effect. Which one you get can make a big difference, and both have their advantages and drawbacks.

The term "half-life" refers to the amount of time it takes for the drug to reach a dosage in the bloodstream equal to half the dosage administered. If a drug has a long half-life, it will still be present in significant doses for as much as twelve hours after being taken. This can lead to a host of problems, especially if you have to get up in the morning and drive on in for that early morning presentation at the office. The drug is still effectively slowing you down and fogging your normal metabolic and brain processes. Your motor co-ordination, your visual perception, and your ability to make correct decisions are all at risk. You are at risk while driving and in any other situation that requires attention, correct judgment, and mental alertness.

These typical after-effects are frequently compounded by our own ambivalence about taking something to get to sleep in the first place. Often we have delayed taking the pill the night before, hoping we might be able to get to sleep in a natural way. We finally give in, take the drug, and fall asleep. But when the alarm goes off in the morning the drug is still present in high dosage, dulling our responses and telling our nervous system to slow down.

The benefits of a long half-life are mostly seen in prolonging sleep; a short-acting drug may wear off too quickly, resulting in early awakening without the ability to fall back asleep. All of these drugs, both short and long in half-life, have a very disturbing effect on REM sleep and deep, delta-wave sleep. It's easy to wake someone up who has been "knocked out" with a benzodiazepene hypnotic. In other words, the sleep we do get is not really very good for us and does not reach the levels needed to genuinely restore brain functions and physiological needs of the body.

Benzodiazepines are also particularly dangerous if mixed with alcohol, especially since someone who combines the two does not necessarily feel intoxicated or more relaxed. *No* sleeping drug, including over-the-counter (OTC) drugs, should *ever* be mixed with alcohol. It's a formula for personal disaster.

Withdrawal from any prescription sleep medication requires careful attention and monitoring by your physician, especially if you have been taking the pills for a period of several weeks or more. If you have been taking medications for a while, you can begin reducing the dosage slowly over a period of time until you are weaned from the drug. You can expect bad dreams, disturbed sleep, irritability, and other unpleasant effects. These can be moderated somewhat with complementary activities, such as the herbal or therapeutic alternatives discussed later on. Established and long-term physical dependency can be very dangerous to your health, even life threatening. You *must* work with a doctor if this is your situation.

Long-acting pills are especially dangerous if you are entering your elder years. As we age our bodies do not process and metabolize drugs as easily. The by-products linger, overwhelming and poisoning the liver and other organs. It's also a bad idea to take drugs when you suffer from apnea. Drugs prolong the period of oxygen deprivation associated with apnea and that's not good news for the patient. You may go to sleep for eternity.

Another population at risk taking sleeping drugs is composed of anyone who is pregnant. That developing baby doesn't need to sleep more—it's already asleep and dreaming most of the time. Benzodiazepines and other drugs disrupt the process, and that can lead to brain damage and abnormalities in the fetus.

To sum up this section, it's best if you can avoid taking any kind of prescription sleeping medication. If you must take one for whatever reasons your doctor determines, then limit yourself to taking the pills for a few days if you can, just enough to try to break the habit of sleeplessness that you have developed. There are better ways to get the sleep you need than resorting to prescription drugs.

OVER-THE-COUNTER DRUGS

Over-the-counter (OTC) sleeping aids are big business in the U.S.—they generate more than $300 million in business a year. A cruise down any supermarket aisle dedicated to "home health care" will quickly reveal shelves stacked with different sleeping medications, some combined with cold medicines or promising help with "flu symptoms." If you take the trouble to read the labels listing ingredients, you will find concoctions that would make Snow White's wicked stepmother take notice as she contemplated her choice of apples. I am personally uncomfortable taking something made up of many unknown chemicals with bizarre names and a host of accompanying warnings. I also don't like the way I feel when I take them, so I no longer turn to them for help.

OTC meds are not really very effective, especially compared to prescription pills, but they may be just enough to allow a break in a pattern of sleeplessness, and that can help you get back to sleep normally. That's especially true when a cold or something similar is helping to keep you awake. Just like their prescription big brothers, though, you need to exercise common sense when taking them. People who take OTC sleep aids get drowsy for the same reason that people who take OTC cold remedies do—the main ingredient will be an antihistamine of some kind, perhaps mixed with an analgesic like ibuprofen to help take the edge off.

Older people and pregnant women should not take OTC pills, for pretty much the same reasons they shouldn't take the prescription variety. OTC pills don't go well with alcohol and can also mess up your motor co-ordination. Taken regularly over a long period of time there are going to be side effects, although it doesn't seem that OTC pills are physically addictive. Next-day grogginess, dryness in the mouth, loss of your mental "edge"—these are common results.

There are lots of people besides old folks and potential mothers who shouldn't take these preparations. Don't give these meds to kids under twelve. If you have an enlarged prostate or urinary problems, don't take them. If you have eye disease, like glaucoma or any kind of breathing problem (asthma or bronchitis), don't take them.

If you are taking one of these OTC preparations regularly, you need to rethink your options. Try going through chapter 2 to see if there are things you can do that will improve your sleeping habits, sleeping environment, or lifestyle. If you have already done all that you can, perhaps it's time to consider seeing a doctor. There is always an underlying reason for chronic, long-term insomnia that needs to be discovered for a true fix. In the long run it's more than worth the temporary extra expense and inconvenience needed to find out exactly what's wrong. Your sleep is key to your entire well-being, and you deserve the best sleep you can get.

NATURAL SLEEP STRATEGIES

In my opinion, there's a better way to go than the over-the-counter route for getting past temporary bouts of sleeplessness. We can develop personal sleep strategies that utilize natural remedies. Some of these, the herbal remedies, have proven themselves over hundreds or even thousands of years. Herbs are certainly not without dangers and pitfalls. Anything that can successfully influence the onset of sleep from the outside is something that deserves our respect. When we intervene to induce sleep we are attempting to alter our body chemistry and nervous functions. That demands our careful consideration.

Herbal formulas and therapies have become widely popular as the cost of health care escalates and people search for ways to deal with their physical problems or ailments on limited budgets. Today, in almost any town of any size in America or Europe, you can find a store dedicated to promoting health-oriented products. These include natural foods, vitamin and mineral supplements, informational books and literature, offers of "alternative" therapies, hormone preparations, herbs and herbal preparations, and much, much more. In the Far East many illnesses and disorders have been treated with herbs for thousands of years.

It's not even necessary to look for a store specializing in health-oriented offerings. As with OTC products, health supplements of every kind have become big business in America, with big corporate dollars behind them. Just walk down that same section or aisle in the supermarket where the cold remedies are, and chances are you'll also come across shelves of vitamins, weight-loss remedies, and herbal "energizers" to perk up your day. The upscale food markets oriented toward organic and "healthy" specialty foods all have supplement shelves, with healthy prices to match. The difference between the upscale store and the chain supermarket products lies in variety, brand name, and, sometimes, quality.

Choose Your Strategy

There are several different ways to trigger sleep using a natural, nonprescription approach of one kind or another. It's up to you to decide which of them, or what combination, might work best for you. Temperament, lifestyle, and personal preferences will dictate your choice. The good news is that there are many different ideas and possibilities to consider. One of them, or a combination of two or more, may be right for you. Broadly speaking, here are your choices for promoting natural sleep:

—— Use supplements of hormones, amino acids, and herbs to stimulate production of the key hormone serotonin, thus calming the brain and initiating the biochemical onset of sleep.

—— Use herbal preparations to calm or sedate the central nervous system, thus encouraging sleep.

—— Use well-established complementary therapies such as massage, acupuncture, acupressure, and other traditional alternative therapies like homeopathy and naturopathy to establish good sleep.

—— Make sure you are in good health through conscious attention to the foods you eat and by exercising your body; support your health with vitamin and mineral supplements, as well.

Let's take these in order and look at what's involved with each one. What are the potentials and possible contraindications for each? How do they differ and how does each approach work?

The Role of Serotonin

Researchers believe that serotonin is one of the keys to sleep. It interacts with other compounds like melatonin and L-tryptophan, telling the brain it's time to sleep. Serotonin is produced by the pineal gland and is a primary chemical neurotransmitter. Neurotransmitters are the biochemical combinations produced in our bodies that send signals back and forth across the enormous numbers of nerve junctions (called synapses) that exist in our bodies. They form the circuit connections between nerve ends and allow transmission of information throughout the nervous system. If there is a deficiency of these chemical compounds, problems result. The nervous system and the brain do not act in the way they are designed. Depression, mental illness, and disease are possible results.

If serotonin levels are low or reduced, or if the serotonin present in the body is reabsorbed too quickly, problems arise. Not only sleep is affected. Other functions that seem to be regulated by serotonin include hunger, mood disorders (depression, feelings of aggressiveness, suicidal thoughts, compulsive behavior), and perception of outer reality.

An entire class of drugs commonly used to treat depression acts to block the reabsorption (reuptake) of serotonin. These drugs are called selective serotonin reuptake inhibitors (SSRIs).

Sleeping Pills, Herbs, and Other Sleep Aids

By inhibiting the breakdown of serotonin (and other neuro-transmitters), SSRIs make it easier for the brain to maintain mood stability. A few popular brand names are Prozac, Paxil, and Zoloft. Unfortunately, for those who take these drugs, one of the common side effects is insomnia, in spite of the increased levels of serotonin. REM sleep and deep, slow-wave sleep are also affected, with all of the undesirable consequences that implies. If you are taking any of these prescription drugs, it's very important not to mix them with any herbal preparations or hormone supplements. It's easy to upset the balance. There is an herb, St. John's wort, which may be a good alternative, but you must speak with your doctor before attempting to switch over to an herbal approach.

If low levels of serotonin cause sleeplessness and depression, why can't we just take a "serotonin" pill and get on with it? Certainly such a pill could be produced with today's technology. The answer lies with something called the blood-brain barrier, which prevents certain compounds from entering the brain directly from the bloodstream. Serotonin is one of those substances. That means that any outside tinkering with the production of serotonin or attempts to regulate time of duration at the nerve endings must be accomplished indirectly. An herb that meets the challenge is St. John's wort.

St. John's Wort

You may have heard of St. John's wort—it is now under serious clinical study by the National Institutes of Health here in the United States and has even become popularly advertised on television as a mood elevator. St. John's wort can help with sleep problems because it acts like prescription antidepressant drugs to block serotonin absorption and reuptake, but without the side effects of insomnia or disrupted REM sleep. Studies show that, in fact, deep sleep periods are increased when St. John's wort is used. This may be a particularly good herb alternative for older folks who are otherwise in good health. The increased levels of serotonin that result from taking St. John's wort help induce sleep. The calming and antidepressant effects of the herb help reduce the kind of sleeplessness caused by worry and concern.

In Europe this common herb is sold in pharmacies and prescribed by physicians. It is used about 70 percent of the time as an alternative to the prescription antidepressant formulas from the drug manufacturers. Unlike the synthetics, the herb doesn't seem to have any significant side effects. Some cases of hypersensitivity to sunlight have been reported. Some researchers caution that it's not a good idea to drink a lot of citrus juices when taking St. John's wort. Before taking it, talk with someone who is knowledgeable about herbs.

One of the real problems with herbal preparations is establishing standardized dosage recommendations. Unlike prescription drugs, there is often a lack of documented clinical trials establishing the optimal dosage for any given herb. This is one of the criticisms frequently leveled against herbal treatments. Fortunately, this is beginning to change, and with a well-researched herb like St. John's wort, there are good guidelines to follow.

Look for a product that has been standardized to 0.3 percent of the active ingredient, hypericin. A typical dosage might be 300 milligrams, three times a day. I am not recommending that dosage here, as everyone is different in body weight, medical history, and unique needs. If you want to take St. John's wort, it's up to you to be responsible and get the kind of specific information needed to determine what the best dose is for you. It will probably take two to four weeks after you begin taking St. John's wort to really notice the effects. In this way it is similar to the brand name SSRIs.

A Word of Caution

This seems like a good place to put in a word of caution about taking supplements to help you sleep. Herbs and hormones are not simply innocuous alternatives to prescription drugs that can be taken as wanted to effect some desired change. Many herbs and hormone supplements are quite powerful, and there can be consequences if they are taken carelessly. There are entire branches of medicine in both the East and the West supported by naturopaths trained in herbal medications and herbal therapies—for sleep and almost everything else.

A little common sense goes a long way when thinking about taking sleep supplements. Don't take any herbs when you are already taking prescription medications or over-the-counter pills. Don't take herbal preparations and drink alcohol. Don't take herbs or other supplements designed to promote sleep if you have to drive or do anything dangerous, like operate machinery or power tools. Never stop taking your prescription pills, and start taking alternative supplements without first consulting your doctor. Especially with sleeping medications, there can be immediate consequences.

Find out everything you can about the herbs or other supplements you are thinking of taking. There is a lot of information right here in this chapter, but you will still need to talk with someone knowledgeable about dosage and frequency. If there is an herbalist or a naturopath in your town, you might consider making an appointment to discuss your sleeping problem.

Today, there is a powerful lobby in the United States that wants to remove herbs, herbal formulas, hormones, and many other supplements from the shelves and restrict public access to these preparations. Supporters of this position cite the lack of clinical studies proving the efficacy of supplements. They ignore many reputable, well-documented, and clinically sound studies that have been done elsewhere, especially in Switzerland and Germany. The anecdotal nature of the claims made for herbs makes many physicians uncomfortable. There have occasionally been false claims made for products, and there are often exaggerated claims for the benefits of any given supplement.

There are documented cases of poor quality control leading to real problems for consumers. One famous example involved the amino acid L-tryptophan.

Sleep Well, Sleep Deep

L-Tryptophan

L-tryptophan is one of the precursors of sleep, part of the bio-chemical chain of events interacting with serotonin. L-tryptophan stimulates the elevation of serotonin levels at the nerve junctions in the brain, thus helping initiate sleep. In 1989 the Food and Drug Administration (FDA) banned this product from nonprescription usage. The FDA position was that L-tryptophan was responsible for a sometimes fatal flu-like disease called eosinophilia-myalgia syndrome (EMS) that affects certain kinds of blood cells. The source of the problem was eventually traced back to contaminated batches of L-tryptophan manufactured by Showa Denko of Japan. Showa Denko wanted to speed up the manufacturing process and used a genetically altered strain of bacteria to accelerate produc-tion. It was not known that this particular strain resulted in pro-duction of a toxic byproduct. Batches of contaminated L-tryptophan were shipped to other manufacturers and packagers, who used them in their preparations. The result was that many different brand names of L-tryptophan were implicated as the source of the illness. The FDA used a blanket approach to remove the products. That was the proper thing to do to protect the public. However, once the true nature of the problem was identified and corrected, the FDA refused to allow the supplement back on the market, claiming that L-tryptophan is a drug.

Prior to this, L-tryptophan was widely available in the United States as an effective sleep aid. It is still fully available without pre-scription in Europe and can be obtained in the U.S. with a prescrip-tion, at prices quite a bit higher than those of the pre-ban days.

Interestingly, in light of the FDA ban on L-tryptophan as a dangerous, sleep-inducing supplement, it is still found as an ingredient in baby formula. Yes, baby formula.

L-tryptophan occurs naturally in many foods. Since it is essential for health but is not synthesized by the body, we have to take it in from outside. The classic source is your mom's old favorite—a glass of warm milk before bed. Other sources include poultry, fish, all milk products like cheese or buttermilk, yogurt, red meats, eggs, and cottage cheese. The body takes what it needs and excretes the rest.

5-HTP

A substitute, 5-HTP, which stands for 5-hydroxy L-tryptophan, can be used for the now-banned L-tryptophan. It is manufactured from an extract of the seeds of *Grafonia*, a type of tree found in Africa. It can also be synthesized. We know that 5-HTP occurs naturally as an intermediate step in the biochemical cascade leading to sleep, between L-tryptophan and serotonin. It is considered to be about ten times as powerful as L-tryptophan, so any supplemental dosage must take this into account. As with all supplements, less can often be better. A good rule of thumb is to start with one milligram per ten pounds of body weight. In a two-hundred-pound adult male, about twenty milligrams can be an effective sleep inducer. Five milligrams might be a better starting point for most of us. Since most commercial preparations come in dosages larger than five milligrams, you may have to break up a tablet or capsule and estimate the lower dosage. This sleep aid is not for kids.

Popular for many years in Europe, in addition to assisting people in sleeping, 5-HTP can reduce appetite if taken about a half hour before meals. But be careful! It's important to make sure you eat lots of protein if you take 5-HTP. Another consideration involves vitamin B_6. Many people take B_6 either by itself or within multiple vitamin supplements. B_6 is one of the vitamins that promote sound sleep. But if it is taken in conjunction with 5-HTP, there could be a problem. It is possible that B_6 greatly enhances the effect of 5-HTP, thus effectively altering the dosage.

One of the side effects of too high a dosage of 5-HTP is mild nausea. The best and safest approach to taking 5-HTP would be to start with a low dosage and observe any effects. You should not take 5-HTP with any prescription drugs, especially with SSRIs like Prozac or Paxil. As with any other supplement, it's not a good idea to take 5-HTP for an extended period. Take it for perhaps two or three months; less is better, and certainly you should take a break after that amount of time. If you want to learn more about 5-HTP, you can search the Internet or find more information at your local bookstore or library. It has become a popular substitute for L-tryptophan. As with every other supplement on the market, try to establish the reputability and quality of the company manufacturing the product. Look for the words "pharmaceutical grade" on the label, as this should ensure a higher quality and attention in the manufacturing process. You may pay a little more, but with supplements like 5-HTP the old adage "you get what you pay for" definitely applies.

Melatonin

Dr. Peretz Lavie, a world-renowned sleep researcher who heads the Technion Sleep Laboratory in Israel, coined the best description for melatonin. He labeled it the "hormone of darkness," because its release is triggered by reduction in light, signaled through the optic nerves. I mentioned melatonin earlier as part of a possible aid to getting over jet lag.

Melatonin is secreted by the pineal gland and is one of the regulators of our circadian rhythms, especially the sleep cycle. Along with sleep benefits, there have been claims that melatonin slows the aging process. Under all the hype is some substance, but there is a lot of disagreement about what exactly the benefits are and what the optimum dosages ought to be.

The antiaging argument is based on clinical studies showing a steady decrease in the production of melatonin from youth to age. Other studies indicate that melatonin also seems to strengthen the immune system. Natural production peaks in adolescence and then steadily declines to about one-half of earlier levels by the time we reach age sixty. It may be a leap of faith to equate melatonin decline with the loss of youth and wishful thinking to hope taking supplemental doses of the hormone might somehow reverse the aging process. All that aside, sound clinical studies verify its role in sleep and sleeplessness.

One of the observable effects of melatonin decline is lighter sleep and less of it. When melatonin is given to older folks in their sixties to their eighties, there is a very significant increase in sleeping time and in the quality of sleep. Melatonin may be a real blessing for older people who simply cannot sleep well or haven't been able to sleep well for years. As with other supplements, if you are considering taking melatonin to help you sleep, some discretion is advisable.

Generally speaking, there is growing evidence that with melatonin a little goes a long way. Many preparations currently on the market offer doses of up to 5 milligrams per capsule. More and more researchers are rethinking dosage and are settling on the idea that very much smaller doses are safer and fully adequate. Personally, I would not take a dose larger than about 0.3–0.5 milligrams. I have tried larger doses and did not like the way I felt. You should always trust the way your body feels. If it lets you know something is not right, go with the feeling. One problem is that you cannot know what your body's natural level of melatonin actually is without very specific tests designed to find out. It's easy to overdo it by adding too much to the hormone mix. Remember—hormones are very powerful substances. Use caution when adding them in as a supplement.

If you can't find a 0.5 or 0.3 dose already made up on the shelf, then buy the 1-milligram size and open the capsule, separating it into thirds. Take one portion, and that should give you about the right dosage. As with everything else, observe how you react to what you take. You can experiment, but starting with less is much better. Side effects can include dizziness, nausea, reduced libido, depression, and weird dreams.

If you have any kind of autoimmune disorder (arthritis, lupus, HIV, etc.), or are pregnant or have bad allergies, don't take it.

HERBS TO HELP YOU SLEEP

We've already talked about St. John's wort, because that particular herb acts directly to influence the production and reuptake of serotonin. There are many other herbs that act differently, mostly to calm and soothe the central nervous system. One of the oldest known and most respected is valerian.

Valerian

Valerian (*Valeriana officinalis*) has been used since early times as a treatment for many different illnesses, particularly any "nervous" condition. Another name for valerian is "all-heal." Valerian has a long and respected track record as a safe and effective herb for any kind of problem that includes anxiety and nervousness. It has been used to treat headaches, fever, pain, arthritis, and menstrual cramps. In the East the Chinese use valerian to treat tobacco addiction and eating disorders, in combination with other herbs. It is the basis for a prescription formula used to treat hyperactive children and has long been used to treat insomnia. Whatever its benefits may be for other problems, it is one of the most successful herbal weapons against sleeplessness and the kind of anxiety that keeps us awake at night. Valerian is the herbal equivalent of several popular tranquilizers sold by prescription only.

Valerian grows well in the summer months and is found in Asia, Europe, and North America. The roots have a peculiar and unpleasant odor. In the first century A.D. the Roman physician Dioscorides is said to have given valerian the name "phu," which ultimately became "phew" in modern usage. Valerian stinks! The odor has been compared to rotten cheese.

Fortunately for us, the preparations available in your local health store don't have the distinctive smell that so inspired Dioscorides. Look for a standardized preparation containing 0.8 percent valerenic acids. Dosage varies according to body weight and need. There have been many well-controlled clinical studies indicating that valerian is an effective sleep aid and calming agent. Of course you must always remember that there is an underlying cause for your sleeplessness, and you must try to eliminate that cause for true relief.

Sleeping Pills, Herbs, and Other Sleep Aids

Unlike prescription sedatives, valerian will not create grogginess or other unpleasant hangover symptoms. It is not addictive. It is potent enough to deserve your respect, and in large doses it can be fatal, just like the synthetic prescription equivalents.

Passionflower

Passionflower gets its name from the resemblance of the flower to the crown of thorns associated with Christ. It is usually sold mixed with other herbs in combinations designed to encourage sleep and stress reduction. Passionflower works to aid sleep by acting as a motor depressant, similar to a narcotic. The herb is calming and has the effect of slightly reducing blood pressure. That makes it a bad bet if you are taking medicine for hypertension. Passionflower has also been traditionally used to help with migraine headaches.

It's a good idea not to try mixing up combinations of herbs (like passionflower and valerian) yourself, unless you are a skilled herbalist. If you should find an unmixed extract of passionflower in your local store, remember this when you are putting together your strategy for better sleep. Don't mix and match without a lot of knowledge and experience.

Kava Kava

Kava kava is another herbal relaxant and is a very good alternative to prescription tranquilizers. As a sleep aid the main benefit comes from reducing anxiety levels, allowing relaxation and the onset of natural sleep. It is frequently used as a pain reliever, helping to reduce muscle pain through its properties as a relaxant.

Kava kava comes from a bush that grows in the South Pacific. Hundreds of generations of island peoples have brewed the herb into a mildly narcotic tea that is still used today in traditional spiritual ceremonies and rituals. You don't have to travel to the South Pacific to get kava kava, although that might be a great way to relax and finally get some sleep (once you get over the jet lag). Every health and herbal store now carries kava kava.

This is an herb that should not be taken by children, if you are pregnant or nursing, if you are driving or operating machinery, or if you are taking prescription drugs or are taking meds for depression—all the same cautions that apply to most of these herbal sleep remedies. The active ingredients in kava kava are called kavalactones, and you should look for a preparation that is standardized to 30 percent kavalactones. Don't take more than 100 milligrams at any one time. It's a good idea to start with less, say 30 milligrams, and increase the dosage if you feel you need it.

Kava kava should not be used for extended periods of time. Large doses will cause dizziness and nausea. Normal doses will produce a feeling of relaxation and well-being, sometimes accompanied by heightened sensory perception. Things may smell stronger, appear sharper, and be heard more clearly. Clinical studies show that kava kava is as effective in reducing anxiety as the benzodiazepines. For sleep, take kava kava about an hour before bedtime. There may be a slight aphrodisiac effect as well, the result of a relaxed body and mind, and heightened senses.

Skullcap

The best skullcap comes from Virginia, where it is popularly known as madweed or mad-dog skullcap. It is supposed to cure hydrophobia in dogs. Skullcap is often found mixed with other herbs in prepared herbal sleep combinations. This one goes well with St. John's wort. The herb acts to calm the central nervous system (it's a relaxant) and has long been considered a restorative as well.

The key to better sleep through herbs, with the exception of St. John's wort, lies in calming the nervous system and relaxing muscular tension that can cause pain and sleeplessness. Herbs help with the "busy mind" syndrome described in chapter 2. Skullcap, like valerian and kava kava, acts to reduce stress. With successful stress reduction comes improved sleep and health, and a restoration of well-being.

Sleeping Pills, Herbs, and Other Sleep Aids

Chamomile

Chamomile is probably the safest of all herbs to use as a calming agent and sleep aid. If you are having bouts of mild insomnia or restlessness when trying to sleep, try a cup of chamomile tea about a half-hour or so before bedtime. There are many commercial preparations of chamomile on the market. You can find this tea everywhere. It is completely non-addictive and has no side effects. The only caution concerns allergies. If you have hay-fever allergies, you may react to chamomile. If you sneeze when you open the box, maybe it's not for you.

Other Herbs

Other herbs are sometimes recommended to help with sleep, either by themselves or in combination. Lavender is said to be calming, but lavender is potentially poisonous if taken internally. Usually it is found in external preparations, like oils and bath salts. The aroma of lavender is frequently found in candles and incense, and it calms the mind. Try a hot bath an hour before bedtime, with a lavender candle or lavender bath salts, and see if this doesn't help you get to sleep.

Lemon verbena has been used to calm the nervous system and makes a good-tasting tea. Hops (but not in beer form) is a helpful component in sleep mixtures.

Used with informed caution and with clear results in mind, herbal sleep remedies are cheap, effective, and safe. The key word here is informed: just taking something that's supposed to help you sleep may not be a good idea. It's up to you to take the trouble to sort out why you are having trouble sleeping and then take the steps needed to really eliminate the root cause of the problem. Once you've done that, there will no longer be a need for sleep aids, of an herbal or any other variety. In the meantime, herbs can help you break the cycle of insomnia and get the rest you need.

COMPLEMENTARY THERAPIES TO SUPPORT SLEEP

The term "alternative," applied to medicine or health-related areas, is like a red flag to many health professionals. There has been a severe backlash in some quarters against traditional medicine over the past years, made worse by the escalating costs of health care and all of the associated problems that go with an increasingly informed population. Just as the traditionalists tend to discount anything that lies outside of their professional training, the alternative folks would sometimes have us believe that anything traditional is tainted either by greed or ignorance.

The truth of the matter is that it is still early in the evolution of our knowledge about health and the mysteries of the mind and body. No one is working with the whole deck. I prefer the term "complementary" when thinking about strategies for personal health that lie outside of the traditional, allopathic mainstream. I think the first person to use the term complementary in this way was Dr. Robert Atkins, who has written several popular books on diet, personal health and well-being. Another well-known advocate of complementary approaches is Dr. Andrew Weil, who frequently lectures and teaches that there are viable and healthy options available for those who do not care to go down the route of prescription drugs and total dependence on their physicians.

Massage, Bodywork, and Body-Oriented Therapies

An excellent strategy for promoting better sleep involves direct touch and intervention with the body. There are many styles, approaches, and disciplines of bodywork. The one you choose depends on your personal preference and needs as well as your physical condition. Body therapies are effective at reducing stress, relieving pain, and even helping with early diagnosis and discovery of potentially disruptive or dangerous physical conditions. A skilled and experienced body person, regardless of the discipline he or she may follow, knows through intuition and training when something is out of kilter.

The most common form of body work is massage, which includes several different methods and approaches. Long a commonly accepted practice in Europe, massage is still growing as a profession in the United States. As a sleep aid, massage can help reduce levels of body tension and promote a sense of relaxation and well-being that sets the stage for peaceful sleep.

The benefits of massage are many. Good, professional massage "gets the kinks out" and leaves the recipient feeling rested and very relaxed. It is a great stress reducer. Swedish massage is the classic form, designed to stimulate circulation and blood flow and improve muscle tone and flexibility, but there are many other styles as well. Possibly the best way to find a massage therapist is by personal recommendation. If you don't know anyone who can point out a good practitioner, open up the phone book.

Legitimate and professional practitioners will be happy to talk with you about what they do, with no financial obligation. You should feel comfortable about working with them before you begin, and you should ask a potential masseur or masseuse about training, style, and experience. Most states have a requirement that massage practitioners be certified according to an approved curriculum, although the amount of training required varies considerably from state to state. Some localities require that massage practitioners be licensed; others have no requirements. The national regulating organization for setting standards of training and professional conduct is the American Massage and Therapy Association (AMTA). Most professional massage therapists will be members of the AMTA. It is necessary to pass a test for membership.

Some body therapies are designed to bring about a deep and permanent shift in the physical body. This can be a good choice if your sleeplessness is being caused by chronic pain resulting from old injuries (sports, accidents), the aftermath of surgery (foot, back, etc.), or just the effects of years of accumulated stress in the body. While massage brings temporary relief, deep therapies are aimed at changing things permanently.

In my opinion the best of all of these is Rolfing. Rolfing is the term used to describe a disciplined and well-thought-out sequence of sessions that can literally give you a new lease on life. Rolf practitioners undergo a very rigorous training and learn to physically manipulate the "soft" connective tissue in the body. By restoring flexibility and movement in the tissue, many improvements in circulation, posture, and ease of movement may be accomplished. Rolfing is not for everyone, but it can be miraculous for some. Many large towns and cities have a Rolfer or two. As with any professional you are considering, talk with the practitioner first and make sure you are comfortable with him or her, and with their training and level of experience. There are sometimes people calling themselves Rolfers who have not actually been trained properly; look for certification from either the Rolf Institute in Boulder, Colorado, or from the Guild for Structural Integration, also in Boulder.

Other powerful forms of bodywork include Hakomi (created by Ron Kurtz), Heller Work (Joseph Heller), Feldenkrais, and the Alexander Technique. Each of these differs in goals, philosophy, and technique, so do your homework. Each has a certifying process requiring disciplined training and commitment. Ask to see the practitioner's certification and ask lots of questions. Expect clear, straightforward answers. If you don't get them, move on. All of these can bring about the kinds of changes needed to support better physical health and better sleep.

Acupuncture and Eastern Medicine

Acupuncture has a tradition dating back thousands of years in the East. In the last few decades there has been a growing awareness of the benefits of acupuncture here in the West, but it is only in the last fifteen years or so that this proven and powerful approach has gained much of a foothold in the United States.

Sleeping Pills, Herbs, and Other Sleep Aids

Traditional acupuncture is based on concepts foreign to Western medical thinking. According to Eastern medical practice, all disease and disorder, including sleep problems, is the result of an imbalance of subtle energies moving throughout the body. This energy (called *chi*, *qi*, or *ki*) moves along well-known pathways within the body called meridians. The acupuncturist uses very fine needles to stimulate different points on the different meridians, according to the diagnosis and training of the practitioner. Simply put, by increasing, decreasing, or balancing energy flow with the stimulation of the needles, health may be restored. There is much, much more to Eastern medical theory and acupuncture, but we don't need to get into that here. If you are really interested, there are many books available with the information you need.

If you can't sleep, an acupuncturist may be able to help you, both in the short term and with whatever the underlying causes of your sleeplessness may be. Frequently acupuncturists will also recommend Chinese and other herbal combinations to support the health and balance of the body. The Eastern herbal philosophy of treatment is different from that in the West, but uses many of the same herbs to achieve the same results. Valerian and skullcap are still the same herbs, for example, even though they may be called by different names and be of a slightly different variety.

If you have never been to an acupuncturist or haven't heard a practitioner of Eastern medicine present a diagnosis and course of treatment, you have an interesting experience in store. To someone who is only familiar with Western medicine, it is like stepping into another reality. There is an interesting aspect to this reality, however: it works. Be prepared to keep an open mind, and remember that this kind of approach has been successful for thousands of years, helping countless numbers of people get a good night's sleep.

Acupuncture is regulated by state licensing boards. An acupuncturist is required to complete a rigorous and thorough curriculum from an accredited teaching institution. There are many schools in the East and a growing number in the West. One of the best schools is in London, another is in Chicago. Several American schools are established and well respected.

Chiropractic

Chiropractic is gaining popularity as health costs escalate and people seek alternatives for maintaining health. There are several different philosophical schools of thought and many teaching colleges of chiropractic. All of them offer extensive training and hands-on practice before certifying their graduates. Chiropractors are regulated by state licensing boards, and there are strict requirements for licensing and certification.

More and more chiropractors include a broad range of alternative approaches in their practices, to compliment the traditional techniques of spinal manipulation that form the core of all chiropractic training. Many employ acupuncture to help their patients, either in the traditional sense, by placing needles, or by using modern electronic devices that stimulate the meridians with an electrical current. They are often knowledgeable about diet and nutrition needs and may be trained in either Eastern or Western herbal medical practices. The best way to find a good chiropractor is to ask around until you get a great recommendation from someone. As with all other practitioners you consider, ask a lot of questions and make sure you feel comfortable with the person you are considering.

NUTRITION, EXERCISE, VITAMINS, AND MINERALS

There have been many books written about diet, exercise, healthful foods, and the role of vitamins and minerals in our bodies. I am not going to try to repeat all of that here. Whatever I say will probably be contradicted by numerous experts anyway, so perhaps we can look at it from the viewpoint of simple common sense and let it go at that.

Sleeping Pills, Herbs, and Other Sleep Aids

It makes sense that certain foods and beverages can interfere with sleep. It doesn't take a genius to figure out that drinking espresso coffee right before bed is probably going to keep us awake. I know people (and perhaps you do as well) who swear that last cup of coffee, not long before bed, relaxes them and helps them sleep. I know one friend who says this, even though for years she has been waking up a couple of hours later unable to easily get back to sleep.

In Europe there is an entertaining and civilized tradition of sidewalk cafés and night life, and it is not unusual to see people drinking strong black coffee late at night. The coffee may be truly delicious and fine, but I'm willing to bet that there is a price in lost sleep that is paid for the momentary pleasures of the cup.

The same is true for alcohol, in all its forms. You may fall asleep quickly, but you will not sleep well or be rested in the morning.

Common sense tells us that beverages containing caffeine, chocolate, or alcohol are going to keep us awake. It also tells us that overeating or eating foods too difficult for our digestive systems to handle easily is also a source of potential trouble. Too much acid in the stomach can ruin sleep, backing up in the classic "acid reflux" effect. Stanley Coren, in his book *The Sleep Thieves*, recommends raising the head of the bed to create a slant toward your feet, preventing the upward flow of acid. That will work, but why not eliminate the cause of the problem, rather than altering one's posture?

Use common sense. You know what foods upset your stomach and your digestion. You may choose to eat them anyway, because they taste good and you love them, but if you can't sleep as a result, perhaps you may want to reconsider your dining choices.

Eating to improve health and stay healthy seems to be a subject of great controversy. You can find a diet and a recommendation for just about any lifestyle or philosophy you wish. Use common sense. Eat some vegetables, don't eat lots of fats and carbohydrates, but don't eliminate them either. Don't believe everything you hear. If you have high cholesterol levels, then eat according to the recommendations of your doctor in a way that will reduce your cholesterol.

Guidelines are not always correct. For example, if you seem to have an allergy to certain grains, why would you follow government recommendations about the proportions of grains in your diet? Use common sense! Try to vary your diet, take it easy on the heavy meats, add in good levels of protein-rich foods like fish and poultry (unless you are a vegetarian—that's another story), and don't overeat. Eat salads, eat fruit if you like (not all fruits are good for all people), drink lots of water (bottled and filtered water is better), and don't chow down before bed or stuff yourself at lunch, and you'll be fine.

If you need to lose weight, don't get crazy about it. Be gentle on yourself, but develop some kind of disciplined approach that will help you lose what you need. Easier said than done, but a little goes a long way when it comes to sleep problems like apnea, in which weight may be a contributing factor. As little as five pounds can make a difference.

Exercise in moderation. Even a walk around the block will help. You don't have to have abs, buns, or anything else of steel unless you really want them. There are plenty of programs and techniques for achieving physical fitness, and a lot of different definitions of what that means. Choose the one that works for you, but choose one.

Vitamins and minerals are an essential component of both physical health and trouble-free sleep. For sleep, vitamin B_6, calcium, magnesium, and niacin are all recommended, but I personally don't think it's a good idea to take your vitamins right before bed—take them in the morning. Probably if you are taking a good multivitamin/mineral supplement, you are getting most of what you need. Calcium and magnesium can be taken about an hour before bedtime. These minerals reduce blood pressure slightly and help to relax the body.

To sum up this chapter, there are many possible ways to alter the body's chemistry and encourage the onset of sleep. They all work, and they all need to be used in an informed and conscious way. You are the one who is in charge of your sleep. Choose the strategy or combination of things that seems to offer you the best chances for better sleep. Try to avoid falling into the trap of relying on either medications or herbs to get you to sleep and keep you there. If you must take something for a while, please consider your alternatives carefully and choose the one with the most potential and least side effects—you'll be glad you did.

CHAPTER SIX

CHILDREN AND SLEEP

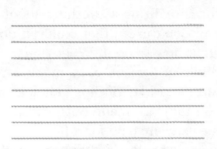

BABIES AND OTHER YOUNG PEOPLE

Ahhh, the sound of a baby's cry. So moving, when we are wide awake and ready to leap into service to our young offspring. So satisfying, when we do whatever is needed to calm our child and the cry turns into contented cooing and gurgling. So frustrating and infuriating, when it's the middle of the night and we are awakened for the second or third time. After a few weeks of this, most parents are wondering how they can endure one more hour, much less any more nights just like the last one. Parental love is certainly a miracle and a mystery, for surely no one would ever survive the first month without it.

There isn't much anyone can do about getting enough sleep during that first month, because baby's digestive system isn't developed enough to permit much more than about two hours between feedings. It isn't possible to establish a longer sleeping pattern until the necessary digestive development takes place. That occurs somewhere around one month of age. Does that mean that your baby could sleep through the night as early as one month? The answer to that is almost, but not quite.

GETTING BABY TO SLEEP THROUGH THE NIGHT

This is a good place to point out something about sleep and infants. There are two key factors that will determine whether or not your baby sleeps through the night. The first factor is physiological—until the physical development needed to keep your baby comfortable is in place, you can forget it. Don't even think about it; just accept that it's in the nature of being a baby. The second factor is realizing something about sleep: sleep is a learned behavior. I don't mean that children don't sleep if they haven't been taught how to do it. What I mean is that how well and how long children sleep is very much a result of choices made by their parents. Many of those choices are made unconsciously, and often they are made out of well-intentioned inexperience. That's especially true for a first child. The whole idea of teaching babies how to sleep is further complicated by a lot of misinformation, especially family traditions passed down from mother to daughter (or son, as the case may be). Family traditions can be deadly, because they may be based on older models of child psychology or misleading ideas passed down from generation to generation (*e.g.*, "When *you* were a baby, I always fed you when you cried. *You* seem to have gotten through it okay.")

The good news for sleep-deprived parents is that it really is possible to establish a peaceful, all-night sleeping pattern in very young children, without much struggle or conflict. Your child's sleep can be peaceful, restful, and serene. More important, perhaps, *your* sleep can be peaceful, restful, and serene. Once you get past the sleep debt built up during that first month or so, you and baby are both going to feel a lot better.

There are lots of things you can do to establish a good sleeping pattern for your baby and for your own sanity. But first things first—you have to wait for that tiny digestive system to get to a point where hunger isn't going to wake your baby up every two hours. How do you know when that has happened? Once you realize it, what do you do then?

Even though every baby is different, if there are no medical or

142

other complications, your baby is going to reach a point in about a month when she sleeps for a period of five or six hours straight. That's the signal to begin changing your behavior toward her. Notice the time frame for this period of lengthened sleep. If she sleeps between 11 P.M. and 4 A.M., make a note of it. After this, don't feed her if she wakes between these hours.

Before this first night of extended sleep, you will have been getting up when she cries and feeding her. Now you have to shift gears. If she wakes and cries during these hours you should comfort her, perhaps pick her up, and then place her back in her crib. Don't play with her, don't wake her up! And don't feed her, because she has already let you know that she can sleep for longer stretches without waking and that she can go that long without food. If you feed her, you are beginning to establish a bad habit: she'll come to expect food every time she wakes, and she won't go back to sleep without it. It's even more complicated, because if she doesn't really need food and you feed her anyway, she will be uncomfortable. We all know what happens when baby is uncomfortable, don't we? Yes, more lost sleep and frustration, plus an unhappy baby to boot.

By avoiding feeding during the magic period of longer sleep, you are establishing the basis for a full, uninterrupted night's sleep. You are building in a pattern of behavior. That pattern will hold unless illness or some other cause disrupts it.

Not being a mother, I'd better be careful what I write here, but almost every mother will tell you that, after a while, she can usually tell what's happening from the particular sound of her baby's cry. Hunger sounds like one thing; "I want attention" like another; pain like another; and so on. It takes time to learn those particular sounds with any new baby. Learning the difference will help you feel more comfortable when baby wakes and cries in the night. It doesn't always mean "I'm hungry."

Often babies (and older children, too—more on them later) will wake and cry out because they are frightened. Sleep is a scary thing for children. What they are really seeking when they wake isn't food; it's safety and security. How you provide that will make a big difference in the results you get.

There have been endless debates over the relative virtues of feeding on a rigid schedule or feeding on an "as needed" basis. Here's the best rule of thumb: *never* wake a sleeping baby, unless it's for medication or some other medical purpose. I don't care if she hasn't eaten in eight hours. When she's hungry, she'll let you know—you can count on it. When you start waking babies up, you are teaching them that sleep is a confusing and disruptive process. How would you like it if someone woke you up at arbitrary times of the day and night, insisting on feeding you when you weren't hungry and generally disturbing your dreams and your comfortable sleep?

When do you like to sleep? Probably at night, unless you are someone who has to work all night. Babies are the same way, or they will be if you teach them the difference between daytime and nighttime. Daytime is for light, for songs, for toys, for noises and sounds, for activities of all kinds. It's a social time, a time to go out in the car, a time to watch things and take in information. Nighttime is for slowing down, for a lessening of the light, for quiet sounds. If you turn your living room into a disco in the evening, don't be surprised if baby can't sleep when you put her to bed.

Part of the underlying problem all parents face is an unconscious one. I'm referring to the assumption that babies instinctively understand the same kind of day and night rhythms we do as adults. If it's dark, we sleep. If it's light, we get up. We take it for granted, and in fact it is built into our circadian cycles. But for babies, it's not that simple. All of the complexities of the nervous system are still in development. It takes about two years for the circadian rhythms to fully establish themselves.

We often make the mistake of projecting our own ideas about things onto our children, forgetting that the way we think and feel about things is very much a function of our life experience and of what we have learned over the years. Babies and children haven't yet learned those things. It's a big mistake to automatically place our preferences over the rhythms and needs of our children. It's an age-old battle, and one that can't be won without heavy casualties. What we can do is adapt, so that everyone gets the sleep they need, along with the quiet time as well.

BEDTIME

Put your baby to bed with consistency. Whether it's at eight, nine, or ten o'clock doesn't matter—that's up to you and your baby's rhythms. What does matter is how you do it, and that you do it pretty much the same way every time. This holds true later on as well, as baby becomes a toddler and then a preschooler. It's a good idea to begin early with a consistent bedtime ritual. Perhaps at as early as two months, perhaps a bit later, make up a consistent set of events that tells her it's time for bed and sleep. A nice bath, putting on her pajamas, a little cuddle time—and then to bed, every time, at the same time.

Try to avoid getting into the habit of putting your baby or very young child to bed when she's already asleep. There's a good reason for this: if she wakes after falling asleep in your arms, it's confusing and unfamiliar. What happened to that nipple? Where's Mom? Where am I? What am I doing here? And the next sound you will hear is—*wwaaahhh!*

With older children it's different. I've found a great trick for getting my almost two-year-old granddaughter to sleep when it's bedtime—she finds it irresistible. I suppose it could be considered a variation on the old idea of singing your baby to sleep. I don't sing, I hum. That's right, I hum at her, in a steady, deep pitch that's fairly monotonous but has a little up and down variety to it. This works for my wife, too. I don't mean that I put my wife to sleep, but that she uses it to put the baby under. It's a great baby-sitting tip, and it will probably work for you also. Just gently hum at her, as deeply as possible in a steady, continuous, relaxing pitch. Make sure there are no other distractions, like the TV or siblings running around. Turn down the lights. In ten minutes or so, she'll be asleep. This can work when you hold her in your arms or when she's in the crib.

145

Sleep Well, Sleep Deep

Barring any medical reasons for waking, most babies will be happily asleep for about twelve hours a night by three months of age, although it could take as long as five or six months for some. I've known parents whose children did not sleep for twelve hours straight until they were two or three years old. It's not uncommon. But that's a terrible period of sleep disruption for both child and parent, and it's usually unnecessary.

You can see from what I've said so far that the real key to peaceful nights with a baby in the house is conscious attention to establishing good sleep habits from the earliest moment possible. The best way not to have a sleep problem with your baby is by preventing one from beginning in the first place. Part of that involves the home environment as well as consistent practices for feeding and bedtime.

Babies are extremely sensitive little people. It's helpful to remember that and think of them in that way. Just as you are disturbed when you get into an argument with someone or when you hear bad news or are upset by some unexpected event, babies also get disturbed when things aren't right at home.

If you are arguing with your spouse, or if you are under an unusual amount of stress and are showing it, your baby will pick up on the "bad vibes" and act accordingly. That usually means screaming and difficulty in sleeping. Of course, if you are arguing and the baby starts screaming, everything gets worse. There isn't anything I can say here that will help to solve whatever it is that may be upsetting you, but try to keep it away from the baby if you can. Use the self-relaxation exercise in chapter 7—it may help.

All of the rules for a good sleep environment given in chapter 2 apply to baby as well. Make the bedroom a pleasant and calm place to be. Every time she goes into the bedroom, it should be a quiet and soothing experience. Leave a night light on—complete darkness is very frightening to babies and youngsters. Make sure the mattress is comfortable and clean. Make sure the temperature is right—not too hot. Put yourself in her shoes (well, booties). See that her nightclothes don't bind or chafe and that she has room to stretch and wiggle as needed. Don't place her on her stomach to sleep, especially during her first year. That's because of the risk of sudden infant death syndrome. SIDS may very well be a kind of sleeping disorder, perhaps like apnea in adults.

When babies cry, they get caught up in the whole process of simply crying. Young children do the same. Peace won't come until you distract them and break the cycle. Get the baby's attention. Get her to look at you and connect with your eyes. Crying seals the baby into her own world, and you need to bring her back out into yours. Then, perhaps, she'll calm down and go back to sleep.

THINGS NOT TO DO AND SACRED COWS

I know that as I sit here and write this, as sure as God made little angels, there are going to be people who think I'm completely wrong about what I'm going to say. There are things parents do and strong ideas they have about babies and sleep that really are no-no's if you want your child to establish a consistent, peaceful sleeping pattern. With few exceptions, all of the things on the list that follows below are in the category of "sacred cows" for many people.

Anything someone who is not the parent says about how a child ought to be raised or treated can stir up trouble. It's always risky to kick a sacred cow, but that's what's needed from time to time. It's up to you to take it or leave it, especially if you are doing something on the following list. There are always exceptions to the rule, so the list isn't perfect. But it should be an exception, not a regular practice. If you are doing any of the things on this list regularly, you are contributing to or causing the very problem you are desperately trying to solve—sleepless nights for you and your child. If you find yourself strongly reacting to something on the list, and if your child has a sleep problem, perhaps you ought to reconsider what you are doing. Here's the list.

Sacred Cows and Other Sleep No-No's for You and Your Child

—— If your child cries, put her in bed with you.

—— If your child cries and wakes during the night, you should always feed her—she must be hungry.

—— If your child cries and wakes during the night, the best thing to do is distract her by playing with her until she's tired and goes back to sleep.

—— If your child won't go to sleep, take her for a drive around the block.

—— If your child wakes up and won't go back to sleep, hold her and rock her until she does.

—— If your child cries at night, you should always pick her up and comfort her.

—— If your child cries and wakes during the night after she's a few months old, you should ignore her—she'll go back to sleep eventually.

—— Children have to learn to adjust to parents' schedules. They should go to bed when it's convenient for me.

—— If she's not going to sleep when she's supposed to, it's because she's just stubborn.

—— It doesn't matter where she falls asleep, as long as she does.

—— She has to learn to grow up—I'm not going to be at her beck and call every time she throws a fit.

—— I've tried everything and there isn't anything I can do. We'll just have to wait until she grows out of it.

Are any of these cows in your herd? If so, let's talk about them and look at each one to see why it might not be a good idea.

If your child cries, put her in bed with you.

Remember, I said at the beginning that there are always exceptions to the rules, so the world isn't going to stop if once in a while your child ends up in the bed. But your sleep will certainly end if you make this into a regular event.

What all of the items on the list have in common is that they all act to teach your baby bad habits about sleep. If you always take her into bed with you, especially if you do this when she wakes and cries, you are in deep doo-doo. Now she has learned that sleep and safety mean being comfortably bounded by a nice warm parent or two. What do you think is going to happen if you decide that enough is enough and it's time for her to learn to sleep in her crib? Yep, either you'd better get a good set of earplugs or learn to sleep curled up in the crib with her. Don't let that happen; don't start in the first place. I know one friend who did and who now stores laundry in the crib, because it's certain that her baby won't sleep there.

If your child cries and wakes during the night, you should always feed her—she must be hungry.

This cow moos very loudly when kicked. It's one of the most insidious of all myths, because it seems to work, at least at first. The baby wakes up and cries, you go in and give her the breast or the bottle, she stops for a bit and may even go back to sleep. After all, that's what you've been doing since she came home. What's wrong with this picture?

What's wrong is that now baby is two, three, four, five

149

months old—or much older—and you are still getting up two or three times a night to feed her and get her back to sleep. You've also noticed that she doesn't really eat a lot and, in fact, gets pretty fussy. Sometimes she doesn't go to sleep for a long time; sometimes she's awake again in minutes. Overall, it seems to be an exhausting and unsatisfying time for both you and the baby.

This is a formula for sleep disaster all around. By appearing with a bottle or breast every time she wakes up and cries, you've taught your baby not to eat well, but to get your attention instead. In fact, she doesn't even need all that food, which will make her grumpy and upset her digestion.

The way out of this is to pay attention and look for that first night when she sleeps for five or six hours at a stretch. That's how you know she's developing nicely and doesn't need to be fed every time she cries. Go into her room, pick her up and soothe her or pat her, talk to her softly for a moment, then put her back to bed and leave. Don't feed her. Don't go back for at least ten minutes if she keeps crying. Keep doing the same thing until she goes to sleep. You will notice major improvement within days, but there is one catch—you have to be consistent. Don't do this twice and then take her into the bedroom with you, or pick her up and head for the rocker. That's the worst thing you can do for everyone's peace of mind, including the baby's.

If you have already been snookered into feeding her every time, you'll just have to break the habit. This is difficult for parents, especially new ones, who are torn by the piteous wails of their deprived and abandoned offspring. And what will the neighbors think? Is this considered child abuse?

No, it's not. It might be abuse of the parents, if babies could be considered abusers, but we can't blame baby—it's our job to teach her how to sleep. Follow the ten-minute regimen above if your baby has already gotten in the habit of crying until you come in and feed her. For the first couple of nights it will be hell, but stick with it. After three or four nights things will change.

I remember seeing a television special some years ago that dealt with exactly this issue—a crying child who wanted his parents to come into the room and give him attention. The parents had established the habit of rocking their child to sleep with a bottle and music when he awoke and cried in the night. Now baby was a toddler, more than a year old, and Mom and Dad had reached the end of their patience with the nightly routine—but nothing else would work. In desperation they called for expert help. I don't remember what expert was called, but the cameras documented the process.

The television crew placed remote cameras in the baby's room and recorded everything that happened. What happened was that when the parents followed the recommended regime (come in briefly and comfort every ten to fifteen minutes, then retreat from the room without feeding or picking the child up) the crying eventually stopped and the child went back to sleep.

At first it wasn't that simple. At first baby carried on as if the world were ending. Then a change appeared—the cameras told the story. It became obvious that he was waking and "hanging out" for a bit before he cried—he wasn't really hungry at all. Next, he would wake up and play for a while before crying. He would rearrange the toys in his crib, giving him a sense of being in control. Finally he would wake up, play for a while, rearrange his toys, and put himself back to sleep, all without crying. It didn't take long for baby to learn that he could put himself to sleep—about five days, although there were a few relapses during the learning process.

What this child really needed to learn was how to put himself to sleep again. Once he understood that his parents were safely nearby and able to respond to him, it became less and less necessary for him to scream for their attention. Because his parents no longer responded by picking him up, feeding him, playing with him, and so on, he learned to entertain himself and eventually to put himself comfortably back to sleep. Your child can do the same.

If your child cries and wakes during the night, the best thing to do is distract her by playing with her until she's tired and goes back to sleep.

Bad idea, folks. It may be fun for baby to have you come in and play with her whenever she wants, but not so good for you and, in fact, not so good for her either. Nighttime is for sleeping, not playing, and that is one of the most basic patterns you must teach your child. Play stimulates and excites. Now baby's wide awake, but it's three in the morning, and you are anything but awake. Your body rhythms are at the absolute bottom, you've got a tiring day tomorrow, and you are mostly asleep anyway—but baby's ready to rock and roll. You want to go back to sleep, but when you try to turn off baby's enthusiasm, you are right back to the old eardrum-shattering protest again. Worse, no one, including baby, gets the sleep that's needed. That means a long and difficult day ahead.

Don't go in and play. You can soothe briefly and retreat. Don't set up a pattern that demands taking on the role of entertainer every night. Unless you're practicing to become the next Jay Leno, it's not a good idea.

If your child won't go to sleep, take her for a drive around the block.

This one's a comedy classic on TV, but it's not funny if you are the one doing the driving. It usually starts when Mom and Dad notice that their little darling falls asleep almost every time they get in the car and go somewhere. Perhaps it's the motion of the vehicle, perhaps the sound of the tires—who knows? All they know is that baby goes to sleep in the car.

Then comes a series of sleepless nights, when nothing seems to quiet her down. Someone remembers the sleep/car thing and, in desperation, they try it. It works! Baby falls asleep! Quiet, blessed quiet, reigns supreme. Dad or Mom returns from their

2 A.M. cruise with a sleeping, cute, peaceful baby in their arms.

If your employer compensates you for the mileage you put on your car, this might be a good idea—you'll make money hand over fist. Otherwise, you'd do better to throw away the keys to the ignition, because you will never get another night of peaceful sleep until this new habit is broken. Taking baby for a ride sets up the conditions under which she'll fall asleep. Once she's figured it out, nothing else will work without a lot of difficulty and upset. You've been warned!

If your child wakes up and won't go back to sleep, hold her and rock her until she does.

This is a little bit like the car solution, except you don't have to drive anywhere. The result will be the same. Once baby gets used to the pleasant motion and close attention of her parent, nothing else will give her the comfort and security she wants. It's a sense of safety that encourages sleep in children. It's scary to slip into the dark nothingness of sleep. It's not going to happen without that sense of security and comfort.

Your challenge is to provide the environment, bedtime patterns of behavior and sense of safety without giving in to your natural instincts to comfort and calm. You may think you are just calming baby down by rocking her to sleep, but you are really teaching her that sleep requires rocking. If you want to regain your normal sleep, don't get into this habit. You'll regret it.

If your child cries at night, you should always pick her up and comfort her.

This one's a little tricky. You're probably thinking to yourself, "Didn't he just say that you should go in and pick her up and comfort her? Is this guy an ogre or something? No rocking, no driving, no feeding, and now I can't even pick her up?"

What I mean by this is that you don't want to get baby into the habit of being picked up and held every time she cries and wakes

153

in the middle of the night. We've already talked about how to come in and comfort her at regular intervals, but that should not usually include picking her up. It's hard, because when you take a look at your hysterical, red-faced, screaming child, your natural instinct is to pick her up and calm her. This is okay when she's very young, but the older she gets the less it becomes a good idea. It's especially hard once she learns to stand; then she reaches out to you with her little arms, tears streaming down her cheeks—you get the picture. Use a little common sense. There isn't a rigid rule about picking her up, but if you do, keep it brief, comfort her, put her back in her crib, and leave the room.

This isn't just for your peace of mind; it's better for her as well. Just like you, she needs her sleep. She's not going to get it while the drama is in progress. You have to lovingly and gently wean her from the habit. Then, as the cameras showed in the example above, she'll learn to relax, play, and go back to sleep on her own. From that time on, you'll know that there is probably a good reason if she wakes up crying and screaming in the middle of the night, like illness or a nightmare.

If, after a few months, your child cries and wakes during the night, you should ignore her—she'll go back to sleep eventually.

This is the other side of running in and picking her up every time she cries. She may indeed go back to sleep eventually, but at a price. The price is an inner sense of safety and well-being that is only provided by reassurance from her parents. If you take this tack and never go in when she cries, you are setting up an environment of insecurity and fear that will come out later in behavioral problems. The idea is not to ignore her needs or desires; the idea is to teach her, with love, how to go to sleep by herself and to feel safe at the same time. All it really requires is a little patience, a clear idea of how you are going to go about it, and an understanding of what the result is that you are seeking. What you are seeking is peaceful nights for you and your baby. How you achieve that is through patient teaching that she is safe and loved. Ignoring her cries is not the right answer. Balance her distress with periodic attention that lets her know you are there and haven't abandoned her. She will learn to calm herself down.

Children have to learn to adjust to adults' schedules. They should go to bed when it's convenient for me.

It seems reasonable that children ought to have a bedtime that allows for some down-time for parents in the evening. What often happens, though, is that as the children grow older it gets harder to co-ordinate it so precisely. An infant or young child can be placed in her crib at a regular hour, but once the circadian rhythms become established, individual sleep patterns begin to assert themselves.

Nap patterns change. Just because it's convenient to have your five-year-old out of the way for an hour or two in the afternoon does not mean she should be taking a nap. Force a nap on her once she no longer needs one, and when it's bedtime she'll be wide-awake. She won't get enough sleep and will be cranky the next day.

Infants sleep up to sixteen hours a day. Toddlers and younger children need about twelve hours of sleep. They can get some of that in naps. Older children, from five or six on, need perhaps ten hours of sleep, and a nap may not be part of it.

The key, once again, is consistent behavior on your part, coupled with gaining an understanding of your child's sleep rhythms. Putting your child to bed at too early a time means that she will lie awake and fuss until she is actually sleepy. Putting her to bed too late will mean she's hard to wake up in the morning and will be cranky and fussy. The right time to put her to bed will have to be determined by trial and error.

Remember "larks" and "owls"? Kids are the same. You may have a little lark *and* owl in your house. If that's the case, putting them to bed at the same time may not be a good idea. Don't force them into synchronization, or there will be conflict.

If she's not going to sleep when she's supposed to, it's because she's just stubborn.

This is a little bit like the last problem. It doesn't take into account the individuality of the child and her sleep needs. Instead the adult arbitrarily decides that it's a question of choice, willpower, and the normal struggle between parents and children for control.

Children don't think like adults. That may seem obvious, but it's awfully easy to forget this, especially as they get older. It's not just a question of them having to learn all of the "adult" things, like going to sleep "when you're supposed to." It's very much a question of neurological development and the formation of all the intricacies of the brain. A child's brain does not develop all of the neurological circuits that will later expand and grow into an adult brain until around age eight. We've all seen children develop through the terrible twos and then into the difficult three-year-old pattern. The growing sense of self as a separate being drives children into temper tantrums and fits as they begin to realize they are not in control. It makes them angry. It makes the parent angry. It can easily turn into a personal battle that neither can win.

If you're wise, you'll try to leave the battlefield behind when it comes to bedtime. All of the suggestions given above, if applied, will probably make this particular issue a moot point. If your child isn't going to sleep when you want her to, it doesn't meant that she's simply being willful. As she grows, her rhythms change, and it's up to you to honor them. Adjust, and don't get caught in a battle of wills. Make it fun and pleasant to go to bed and time it to her natural need for sleep—then you won't have much of a problem.

It doesn't matter where she falls asleep, as long as she does.

This was mentioned briefly earlier. It does matter, unless you're in one of those situations where you're not at home and it's time for a nap. Going off on a family expedition for the day will probably find your kids asleep but not in bed sooner or later. That's okay. I'm referring to when you are at home. If your little girl gets in the habit of falling asleep on your shoulder while you watch television, you're teaching her a bad way to sleep. It's always the same: good sleep habits demand consistency. The consistency you provide for your child will establish how the sleep pattern looks. If it's consistently not in her bed, she'll consistently want to fall asleep somewhere else and have trouble when you try to put her in her crib. Avoid this before it ever gets started.

She has to learn to grow up—I'm not going to be at her beck and call every time she throws a fit.

There's not a lot to say about this—it's similar to some of the others. Babies, toddlers, young children, and older children are not "grown up" by definition. They're not going to "grow up" because we want them to. If your child is throwing a fit, it's for a reason, not because she simply wants to bug you. If she's screaming and crying during the night, you have to do something about it, and not just for your own peace of mind. Almost always, if there is no medical complication, you are looking at a sense of insecurity or fear in the child. Try the things mentioned throughout this book, and you will be rewarded with peaceful nights and a happier child.

I've tried everything and there isn't anything I can do. We'll just have to wait until she grows out of it.

I hope that by the time you have reached this point, you realize that this statement doesn't make a lot of sense. There's always something you can do that you haven't tried. If you have actually tried everything already mentioned without results, something is probably wrong. Make sure there isn't a medical reason for a sleep problem. For example, a "colicky" baby will fuss and scream because of the discomfort. A little chamomile tea may help, or a change in formula. Perhaps there's an allergy to milk or some other factor. Talk with your doctor. Be patient and keep calm, and it will all work out.

Sleep is dependent on so many different factors that you need to make sure you have addressed them all. Don't give up. Most sleeping problems for babies and youngsters can be handled by following the guidelines above. Occasionally, there might be a sleep disorder causing the problem, just as with adults.

SLEEPING PROBLEMS AND DISORDERS IN CHILDREN

Diagnosing a sleep disorder in a child can be difficult. If you suspect that your child may have one of the sleep disorders described below, check it out with your doctor. Some of these respond well to the tips given below. Others, like narcolepsy, require medical treatment.

Bed-Wetting (Enuresis)

Bed-wetting is a normal occurrence for children up to about age five. After five years of age it may signal some underlying problem. Causes can be either physical or psychological. For example, a child who is very insecure or emotionally sensitive may tend to wet the bed long after others have stopped.

The real challenge is to remain patient and to not place blame on the child for failing to have bladder control. Make sure there is no physical cause at the root of the problem that needs to be addressed, like a bladder infection. Talk with your doctor or another health care professional about how you might help your child get through the problem. You may have to pay close attention for a while and make an effort to teach your child better control. There's a right way and a wrong way to do this, so make sure you have sought professional advice about how to do it.

Children often confuse dreams with reality. It is not uncommon for a child to dream of getting up and going to the bathroom and urinating, only to find in the morning that it really was a dream. A dream seems completely real to a child, and it's important to remember this. She's not doing it on purpose.

Avoid drinks before bedtime. For at least two hours before bed, don't give your child anything to drink except, at most, a sip of water. Make sure he or she goes to the bathroom before getting into bed. Avoid soft drinks and the like at dinner. Soon enough, things will be dry and comfortable.

Narcolepsy

This disorder is serious and must be treated by a physician. Just as with adults, a child can suddenly fall asleep in the midst of other activities. Attacks occur without warning: one moment the child is present and active, the next sound asleep.

Narcolepsy has nothing to do with the amount of sleep your child is getting, although it will get worse if much of a sleep debt is built up. It seems to be a genetically linked disorder; if you or someone else in your family suffers from narcolepsy, be aware that your child may also be at risk. If your child is especially hard to wake up in the morning and is confused or angry when woken, that might be a sign of narcolepsy, along with other symptoms. It could also just be a sign of sleep deprivation, so don't jump to conclusions.

Naps may help, but you still need to see a doctor.

Sleepwalking

Sleepwalking is far more common in children than in adults. While adult sleepwalking is a very serious problem, children will probably outgrow it with time. Usually sleepwalking occurs in children about four to eight years old. As with adults, kids don't know they are asleep and you should not wake them. Simply guide them back to bed, or help them lie down again under the covers.

159

The main concern for children is protecting them from harming themselves accidentally while asleep. If you have a child who sleepwalks, make sure that he or she can't fall down stairs or trip on something. Set up a simple alarm system to alert you, perhaps a noisemaker on the child's bedroom door; keep windows closed and locked. If the sleepwalking continues over a long period of time, see your doctor.

Apnea

The same causes of apnea given in chapter 3 apply to children. The same types may be found, with the most usual involving some sort of obstruction of the upper airway. The symptoms are similar: loud snoring, headaches, dullness, and disturbed sleep. With children, the cause may be a simple infection of the respiratory tract—kids are always getting something, as we know too well. Sometimes the child might be sleeping in an awkward position. Changing the position will cure the blockage.

Swollen tonsils and adenoids can also cause obstruction. A physician can determine if this is the cause, and removal or reduction of the swelling will eliminate the apnea.

Apnea in children can be subtle and very dangerous. A consistent lack of oxygen caused by apnea results in developmental retardation, especially in the brain. Before doctors understood the effects and even the diagnosis of apnea, severe difficulties were encountered with children who had the disorder. If you think your child has apnea, please see your physician. It's critical for your child's health.

Nightmares and Night Terrors

Nightmares are common at any age and are especially frequent from ages three to six. Often the child dreams of being chased by nameless and ill-defined monsters. It's a normal stage of development. Children of this age are becoming more and more aware of the enormous complexity of the world. For the child, it's a world not under personal control. It's a very large world, full of rules, warnings, incomprehensible actions, and events that are difficult to understand and integrate into the child's experience. The brain becomes overwhelmed and overstimulated. The result is a nightmare.

The way to deal with nightmares is to acknowledge how scary they are and to let the child talk it out. You can say it isn't real, but don't be surprised if your statement is met with skepticism or disbelief. To the child it is very real, and children don't know how to separate dreams from reality. Some people think you can teach children to not be scared and to fight back in the dream. I think it's okay to tell a child to kick the monster or punch it in the eye. You can also tell your child to just call out for Mommy or Daddy in the dream. You want to encourage a sense of control, with the idea that it's actually possible to fend off the monsters if they show up. But don't get too far out with this. Children are not really capable of learning how to control dreams, nor should they try to learn how. They are too young, and dreams have much to teach them down the road. Years of working with dreams have convinced me of this.

Night terrors are different from nightmares and often occur when children are drifting off to sleep. Perhaps it's associated with the sense of falling into darkness: some children will actively resist falling asleep because of that feeling. Generally, the child will scream and appear to be awake, but in actuality will be asleep. If awakened the child will typically be confused. One thing that can help prevent night terrors is the old traditional stuffed toy. Giving a young child a soft, stuffed friend helps ease the transition from parent to bed and the darkness of sleep. The toy is a kind of bridge between the known and the unknown. Try it if your young child is having night terrors. Add in a lot of love and reassurance, and the terrors will pass sooner or later.

Headbanging

Don't worry too much about this unless it is quite severe. Very disturbed or autistic children can engage in serious headbanging and rocking back and forth, but usually that is not what's going on. It should stop by age three or four, and should never be hard enough to injure your child. If you suspect something more intense, speak with your physician.

Confusional Arousal

This is the name given to a disorder that looks exactly as it sounds. The child seems to wake up, may actually be waking up, but is confused and disoriented, upset and inconsolable. It will take a while before the child is truly awake. Usually such an event occurs during the night, and the child will return to sleep when it is over. It's a common problem and not cause for undue concern. It will disappear as the child matures.

Adolescent Sleep Needs

Everyone who has had a teenager around the house knows that previous sleeping patterns go out the window with the onset of adolescence. Usually it looks like excessive sleepiness during the day and a pattern of staying up late at night. Studies indicate that teens still need ten hours of sleep a day. Most aren't getting that much. Most adolescents are wandering around sleep deprived. Where the deprivation shows up is during the school day.

It's one thing to be out with friends having a good time or hanging out on the Internet at one in the morning. It's another, as far as motivation and interest goes, to pay attention in boring classes about subjects that appear to have no relevance or value for your life. A lot of teenage inattention in school can be laid at the doorstep of sleep deprivation, all other things being equal. When we are sleep deprived, all it takes is one dull class and we're off to a never-never land that is not quite sleep and is certainly not wakefulness. It is also not very good for learning anything.

How can you deal with it? Rules about bedtime can handle part of it—be flexible and allow as much freedom as seems reasonable to you, consistent with creating a framework for enough sleep. Be aware that some studies show teenagers' biological clocks get out of sync with the rest of us. This might just be a case of delayed sleep-phase syndrome (DSPS), caused by staying up late and going to bed later, or it may actually be inherent in the physiology of adolescence. If it's inherent, we have to live with it. If it's DSPS, then it can be shifted by gradually readjusting the hours for sleeping, just as with a night-shift worker or some other situation where the biological clock has gotten out of adjustment. If you are trying to adjust your teen, good luck!

Children, adolescents, and adults all have one thing in common: we all need enough sleep. Up to our first year, we need about sixteen hours of sleep, sometimes as much as eighteen, to maintain neural development and health. Gradually, the amount decreases, to about fourteen hours with toddlers and young children, about ten or eleven hours for a five-year old, and about ten hours for children up to age ten or eleven. It stays around ten hours right up to about twenty years of age. Then it drops to an average of eight for younger adults.

One of the best things you can do for your children is to make sure they get enough sleep and to give them the sense of security and safety that will help them to sleep peacefully. It's not automatic; we have to work at it. But it's really not a lot of work, and well worth the reward of having healthy and happy kids.

CHAPTER SEVEN

SELF-HYPNOSIS FOR SLEEP AND WELL-BEING

. . . hypnotized, mesmerized, by what my eyes have seen . . .
—Natalie Merchant

ALL ABOUT HYPNOSIS

Hypnosis is one of those subjects that everyone has heard about, but almost no one seems to understand when you ask them to describe it. Most of our exposure to hypnosis has been through stage hypnotists or Hollywood dramas portraying dark-eyed and sinister men using hypnosis for evil purposes. Stage hypnotists are performers who entertain by hypnotizing volunteers and then asking them to engage in various silly actions, to the great amusement of the audience. They also usually do something to demonstrate the mysterious powers of the human mind, turning laughter to wonder. Movie hypnotists usually bear no resemblance to the real thing and are most often figments of a scriptwriter's fertile imagination.

I remember being taken to see a stage hypnotist when I was about eight years old. After some preliminary remarks, the hypnotist began a group induction to find suitable subjects in the audience, who would come up on stage and participate in the act. This simply meant that he began speaking and suggesting various images and actions, asking people to close their eyes and requesting cooperation from the audience. I was fascinated and wanted very much to be a subject, but being only eight, I could not resist the temptation to open one eye from time to time to see what was happening with the rest of the audience. Needless to say I was not hypnotized, but several people clearly were.

I never forgot that evening. People clucked like chickens, tried to sit down in chairs that were already occupied, and thought they had suddenly lost all their clothes. Others barked like dogs instead of speaking and even became so completely rigid that the hypnotist could stand on them while they were stretched across two chairs. Amazing!

I didn't know it at the time, but I had just been introduced to a fundamental and mysterious truth about our human nature: the subconscious mind has almost unbelievable power to affect our body and our well-being. If we can be hypnotized to cluck like a chicken or to allow a two-hundred-pound man to stand on us without problems, what else is possible? The answer is quite a lot. One of those possibilities is using hypnosis to help us sleep.

Hypnosis has an interesting history, filled with colorful characters of all sorts. This hasn't helped its reputation as a legitimate form of therapeutic intervention. Sometimes people have used hypnosis for their own doubtful ends. Perhaps the best known example is the monk Rasputin. He used hypnosis to stop the hemophilic bleeding of the Russian czar and czarina's son, Alexis, during the rule of the last Russian czar. Hypnosis can indeed stop or slow bleeding and can be used in this way to support surgical procedures. In Russia at the time, this seemed to be magic to most people and probably black magic at that. Rasputin's strange and arrogant personal presence, crude habits, and blatant sexual behavior, along with his enormous influence on the czarina, contributed to the underlying public discontent that ultimately led to the Russian Revolution and the deaths of the Romanovs.

The first man in recorded times to become famous for taking

people into a hypnotic state was Franz Anton Mesmer, who died in 1815. You may have heard of the term "mesmerism," which described his work. "Mesmerized" has sometimes been used instead of hypnotized, but it really isn't the same thing. In fact, Mesmer had no idea how he was achieving his results, thinking that they were due to an elaborate combination of "magnetic fluids" in the body and the alignment of the "heavenly bodies." While making mysterious passes with his hands in front of his subjects, he used magnets and baths full of iron filings to attempt his cures.

Mesmer lived in Vienna and Paris and seems to have been a combination of genuine healer and accomplished con man at the same time. Mesmer called his work "animal magnetism." He was the rage of the aristocratic and wealthy salon circuit in Paris prior to the French Revolution of 1789. He attempted to prove the validity of his work to a committee of scientists, including Benjamin Franklin, but was discredited. Whatever the merits of his unproven theories, Mesmer unknowingly induced hypnotic trances in his subjects, thereby effecting some interesting and sometimes miraculous cures, particularly for what we would now call "stress-related disorders."

The word "hypnosis" is a compliment to our old friend Hypnos, the Greek god of sleep. It was coined by a man named James Braid, an English physician who lived mostly in the first part of the nineteenth century. Dr. Braid mistakenly thought that hypnosis was a form of sleep. When he realized his mistake, he made a valiant effort to change the name, but it was too late—the word "hypnosis" had become the accepted description of whatever it was that was happening.

What was actually happening is still a subject for debate, even today. The best definition I have heard for hypnosis is that it is a state of deep relaxation and heightened suggestibility. The recognition and use of the power of suggestion as a therapeutic tool was made popular by another doctor, Emile Coué. Coué is famous for his suggestion that "Every day, in every way, I am getting better and better." He used hypnosis and suggestion with his patients to effect improvement. Coué formulated several "laws of suggestion" and eventually stopped using hypnosis in favor of the positive affirmations and suggestions he developed. Today, modern hypnotists have gone back to combining the two, with powerful effect.

The man most responsible for establishing psychological and medical respectability for the use of hypnosis was Milton Erickson. Dr. Erickson was an interesting and innovative man, some would say a genius. One of his most powerful ideas was that each of us contains all of the resources we need within ourselves to accomplish any desired change. The role of the hypnotherapist thus becomes one of helping the client organize and evoke that change.

The problem with pinning down the hypnotic state is that we are dealing with the subtleties of consciousness. No one actually understands what consciousness is. That's why we have to settle for recordings of brain waves and other neurophysiological measurements in an effort to create a scientific framework for understanding. The exact mechanism and nature of the hypnotic state will probably never be known, but the effects can be demonstrated and repeated.

There are many false ideas about hypnosis. Probably the biggest one is that we can be forced to do something against our will if we are hypnotized. No one can be forced to do something under hypnosis without giving permission. A hypnotist can suggest, but not compel. The nature of the person determines the nature of what he or she will do when hypnotized. Hypnosis is a dance of cooperation between the therapist and the client.

The best hypnotist in the world cannot induce a hypnotic state in someone who is not willing to be hypnotized. It's also true that hypnosis is not sleep, as Dr. Braid eventually discovered. Most people are completely aware of everything that is happening when hypnotized and are perfectly capable of getting up and ending a session at any time. Under hypnosis you are alert and relaxed, not asleep. The famous "Sleep . . . sleep . . . you are going to sleep . . ." of Hollywood movies is not how it's done.

But poor sleep is definitely one of the things that can be helped by using hypnosis.

It's easy to resist being hypnotized. The techniques given in this chapter for self-hypnosis and sleep will work to the degree that you choose to allow them to work. If you are concerned about hypnosis or feel uncomfortable with it for some reason, then you may wish to skip ahead to chapter 8. But if you are willing to try some tested and well-proven techniques for self-hypnosis and relaxation, then this chapter is for you.

Self-hypnosis is nothing new—in fact, all of us spend some part of our day in a state of self-hypnosis. If you don't believe me, think about it for a moment. Have you ever driven to work or some other familiar place, only to arrive at your destination without actually recalling the details of the trip and how you got there? Or perhaps you were watching television and suddenly realized that twenty minutes went by—without a clue about what you've been watching! I could go on giving examples of minutes or even hours when you were simply not consciously paying attention to what you were doing, yet things were going on just the same. Time passed, something happened, and you don't recall the details—that's self-hypnosis.

Perhaps you have spent some time thinking about something, visualizing it in your mind's eye, imagining how that new carpet might look or how the project is going to turn out. You open your eyes and go on with your day. That was an example of self-hypnosis. Self-hypnosis is a natural state, and we all have a lot of practice in doing it, so it will be easy for you to use it to help you sleep.

One of the keys to sleep is relaxation, since a tense and active body will not easily allow sleep to come. Any techniques for promoting sleep have to take this into account. The first step in self-hypnosis is learning how to consciously relax. The techniques for self-hypnosis that I am going to present here are based on my experience and on a simple process developed by the National Guild of Hypnotists, one of the principle certifying and teaching bodies for hypnotherapists in the United States.

SELF-HYPNOSIS FOR RELAXATION AND STRESS RELIEF

Just like anything else we do, our environment has an impact on our experience. This exercise in relaxation can be done anywhere (except behind the wheel!), but it's going to be easier to master if you first learn it in a calm and quiet setting. I always begin a session by asking my clients to get comfortable, and you should do the same. Pick a comfortable chair or couch, or lie down if you like. I prefer to sit comfortably.

Make sure that you will not be interrupted. Unplug the phone, make sure the cat won't jump in your lap or that the baby's asleep—whatever it takes. It's only for a few minutes, so it shouldn't interrupt your normal routine to any great degree. Take off your glasses, if you wear them.

One of the most powerful and natural tools we have for relaxation and health is found in the breath, so we will use breath as a way to begin our exercise.

Relaxation Exercise and Visualization

—— After you have picked your spot for comfort and quiet, begin to gently focus your attention on something in front of you—a spot on the wall works really well. Let your head and shoulders be comfortable and your eyes level.

—— You are going to take three slow, deep breaths. Breathe in as fully and deeply as you can, without straining or trying for that extra bit. As you reach the end of your third breath, hold for an extra few seconds and then exhale slowly. As you exhale, close your eyes. Relax and let the tension drain out of your body as you exhale.

—— In your mind's eye, imagine the number twenty-five. You can choose any color for the number or the back-

170

ground. Gold against black, blue against white, red against gold—it doesn't matter. If you prefer, you may see the number written on a blackboard or displayed on a computer screen. Whatever works for you.

—— Beginning with the number twenty-five, slowly count backward to the number one. Each time, see the next number against the background you have chosen. If you have trouble visualizing, don't worry—just do the best you can and slowly go on to the next number, counting backward until you reach the number one.

—— When you reach the number one, pause for a beat; then count forward from one to three. When you reach the number three, open your eyes. You will feel relaxed and refreshed.

—— Practice this exercise twice a day for at least a week before going on to the other steps given below.

This is a great way to replenish your batteries during the day, and it has the benefit of only taking a few minutes. Can't get things to quiet down at your desk at work? Take a brief trip to the restroom, go into a stall, and ––relax! Got a busy day at home and feeling a little frantic and rushed? Sit down where it's quiet, focus, and breathe, count backward for two or three minutes, and—relax! About to go in and take that big test or make that presentation? Use this technique to calm and center yourself so you'll be at your best.

Practice this exercise every day, twice a day, for a week. It does more than help you relax—you are teaching yourself to enter a light, self-induced hypnotic state that can be used for many things, including sleep. The next step to helping yourself sleep is to combine this with positive suggestions that you will give yourself at the end of the day.

I'd like to point out something here. Although the techniques presented here are geared toward helping you sleep, they can work equally well to help you prepare yourself for success, relax and reduce stress, or assist you with some specific goal or objective that you would like to accomplish. The reason for this is that the mind doesn't much care how you use hypnosis to accomplish something. If you want it to happen, being in a light state of hypnosis simply makes it easier and helps your subconscious mind support you in achieving the goal. If the goal is sleep, fine. If it's losing weight or becoming more prosperous, it's equally fine. The mind doesn't care. You can adapt the ideas here to suit your particular needs. I encourage you to do so.

The next step in getting to sleep is reprogramming yourself with positive suggestion. In the proven tradition of Dr. Coué you can tell yourself something positive and beneficial. Continue to practice the relaxation exercise twice every day while you add in the pre-sleep exercise below.

Giving Yourself a Hypnotic Suggestion

—— As you lie in bed, rest your hands gently on the center of your chest.

—— Make sure you are comfortable and relaxed. If you like, you can use the self-relaxation technique given earlier.

—— Choose a suggestion to give yourself about sleep. For example, you might say to yourself something like "Tonight I will sleep deeply and peacefully and wake up feeling great in the morning," or "It's easy and comfortable for me to relax and sleep." You get the idea. Make up something short, direct, believable, strong, and positive. It's important that you believe that what you are suggesting to yourself can actually happen. Your suggestion sums up what you are trying to do.

—— Say this phrase ten times to yourself slowly in your mind or out loud, with your eyes closed, gently pressing your fingers into your chest each time you say it. This helps anchor the suggestion in your physical body. Then repeat the phrase to yourself again three to five times, without pressing down.

What you are doing by going through the pre-sleep suggestion technique is teaching yourself what it is that you need to learn or do. Trust me, it can work for you. It might take a few days or even longer, but give it a chance. There is still a third step in our self-hypnosis learning that can really help things along and increase your success.

So far you have learned to relax, by breathing and visualizing, and you have learned to begin teaching yourself through positive suggestion. What remains is to combine the two.

Getting Better Sleep by Combining Relaxation and Positive Suggestion

—— Get a blank three-by-five-inch index card and write down your positive suggestion about sleep. Your suggestion needs to be more than just positive; make sure it's simple and clear. Especially make sure that it is believable. It's probably not believable to tell yourself that you are going to go to sleep at ten and wake up at six, every day, without fail, especially if you haven't been able to go to sleep at ten since you were fourteen years old. Make it realistic and something you can believe in.

—— Carry this card with you wherever you go. Take it out and read it from time to time, and use it in the rest of the exercise, as given below.

—— Find a quiet and comfortable spot to sit and relax, just as in the earlier relaxation exercise. Make sure you are comfortable and that you will not be disturbed.

—— Focusing first on the wall as you did before, take out your card and hold it in front of you; now you are focusing on the card and the suggestion you have written on it. Imagine yourself doing whatever it is you have written. As much as possible, feel and see the result you desire—better sleep, peaceful sleep, undisturbed sleep—whatever it is.

—— When you have read the card and visualized the result in your mind's eye, let the card slip out of your fingers and take a deep breath, just as you did when practicing the relaxation exercise. Exhale, breathe again, exhale, breathe again, and close your eyes. Hold the breath for a beat, and then relax and let go as you exhale. Allow yourself to enter a state of deep relaxation (hypnosis).

—— Instead of counting backward from twenty-five to one, as you did before, let the suggestion you have written on your card repeat itself over and over. In your mind's eye, see yourself accomplishing the suggestion—sleeping peacefully, awakening refreshed and fully rested—whatever it is you've told yourself you want to do.

—— Do not be concerned about doing this visualization perfectly. It's okay to let the words of the suggestion break up or to not get it exactly right. It's okay if you can't perfectly visualize the result. Just relax and take what you get, bringing your attention back if it wanders.

—— In a few minutes you will feel that you've done enough. At that point, count forward from one to three and open your eyes. You will feel refreshed and relaxed.

Do this twice a day for at least two weeks and keep doing it as long as you wish. That's all there is to it! Be patient and give the technique time to work. You are teaching yourself to sleep differently, to act differently, and it can take time. Combine this with giving yourself the same suggestion at night, and you will soon be sleeping much better than before.

You can use this technique of auto-suggestion and self-hypnosis to help effect change in any area of your life. For example, if you are overweight and want to lose a few pounds, try self-hypnosis. Remember that any suggestion must be realistic and believable. It may not be realistic for you to quickly lose fifty pounds, but it is certainly realistic to lose five. Once you've lost five, then you can lose five more, and so on.

It's important to acknowledge yourself when you succeed in achieving any part of your goal, even if it's not perfect or exactly what you want. Suppose you are able to improve your sleep. Perhaps you still aren't getting all of the sleep you need, but things are getting better. Don't ignore it and decide the technique isn't working. Perhaps you set your expectations too high, or maybe you're not following the directions exactly. Notice the improvement you do get, congratulate yourself for succeeding to some degree, and keep after it; you'll get there. It helps to cultivate an "attitude of gratitude" for the results that you do get. Be thankful that things are changing for you in the way that you want.

Another useful thing you can do to support yourself in getting more sleep is to record your suggestions and listen to the tape every day. You don't need to try for a Grammy award when you are making your recording. It's easy. Here's how to go about it:

Making Your Own Tape of Positive Suggestions for Sleep

—— Get an audiocassette recorder and a fresh cassette. I prefer full-size cassettes to the mini variety, as the quality tends to be better, and they are easily duplicated, if necessary.

—— Select a piece of background music for your recording. It should be something peaceful and calming, without vocals. Music is not necessary, but I have found that it does add something to the mix that is helpful.

—— Write down your positive suggestions about sleep. Make up more than one—at least two or three. You don't need eight or ten, though. Keep them simple, direct, and believable.

—— Practice saying the suggestions you've written out loud, until you are comfortable repeating them. Try for an even and steady rhythm in your voice. Remember that you are going to record these for your own use only, to send a message of peaceful relaxation from yourself to yourself. Put a little love in your voice. You are the beneficiary, if you do.

—— When you are comfortable with the words and phrases, start the background music, not too loud, and begin recording your suggestions. Repeat each suggestion several times, with a pause between each one. Talk gently and calmly to yourself, putting your belief and desire into the words. Work your way slowly through the list you've made—you have as much time as you need.

—— When you have gone through each suggestion several times, return to the first suggestion and repeat it again a few more times. If you like, you can go through the entire list again, but it's not necessary. Play with it and have fun. What you are doing is teaching yourself how to have a good night's sleep.

—— Let the tape end with the music playing in the background. You can gradually lower the volume of the music if you wish, until it fades away.

—— Listen to the tape through earphones periodically to re-enforce your new self-programming for better sleep. Don't use it when you are driving or doing something that requires attention! You can put on the tape at night when you get into bed, if you like. You may find that you are asleep before you reach the end.

Self-hypnosis is mostly about relaxation, practice, and your desire to get a result. Since you are the only one who is doing the hypnotizing, you needn't be concerned about what anyone else is doing or about what they may think. You are free to create and explore. Self-hypnosis can open the gateway to the power of your mind to affect your body and your well-being, and that is no small thing. Try it, and you may be sleeping better than ever before in just a few weeks.

CHAPTER EIGHT

SWEET SLEEP

. . . the innocent sleep, Sleep that knits
up the ravell'd sleave of care . . .
—Shakepeare, *Macbeth:* Act II, Scene II

*S*hakespeare's famous words have never been equaled when describing the essence of sleep. The rest of the quotation goes on to list more benefits of sleep, but these few words say it all. Sleep is the restorer, the healer, the soother, one of the few things that can make the difference between a life well lived and one that is a living hell. We can have all the money we need, people in our lives who love us, work that satisfies us, and everything that life offers—but it will all taste like dust and ashes if we cannot get enough sleep to enjoy it. Our health, our vitality, our joy of life are all keyed into sleep. Sleep is critical to our well-being. Sleep is so intricately woven into our existence that it cannot be separated from any aspect of our lives.

A lot of different ideas have been presented in this book about what sleep is and how to do something about it if we are not sleeping as well as we would like. By now you should have a clear picture of why you are having trouble sleeping. Perhaps you have applied some of the ideas given earlier and are already sleeping better. If not, this seems like a good place to bring everything together and lay out a simple plan for improving your sleep, and therefore improving your health and sense of well-being.

THREE STEPS TOWARD BETTER SLEEP

Simply put, there's a three-step process to better sleep. The first step is to identify the nature of the problem: what is the reason you are not sleeping well? The second step is to make a plan to bring about the needed changes, so sleep can return. The third step is to implement the plan, modify it as needed, and carry it through to completion.

Step One: Identify the Nature and Cause of Your Sleep Problem

To help you pin this down I've created a simple series of statements below. These are different from the "sleep potential" inventory given in chapter 2. The sleep potential inventory should have given you a clear picture of the many different factors affecting your sleep. This is a good time to review the results, before you go any further, or you can refer back to it as we go along.

What we want to get to with these new statements is something a little different: we want a kind of snapshot of your knowledge about sleep and sleeping. It is knowledge that will solve the problem for you—nothing else will do. You've heard of "street smarts." This is "sleep smarts," not quite the same thing but close enough. Respond to the statements below with a simple "yes" or "no." There is no correct response. You simply want to understand the nature and cause of your sleeping problem.

Sleep Smarts Questionnaire

—— I have made all the needed adjustments in my sleeping environment that can help me sleep better.

—— I understand the relationship of alcohol, nicotine, and caffeine to the quality of my sleep.

—— I understand the relationship of my eating habits and food preferences to the quality of my sleep.

—— I understand how circadian rhythms affect my sleep.

—— I think it's important to make enough time in my day to get a full eight hours of sleep.

—— I make sure that I take time to relax and let go of daily problems and worries.

—— I take prescription medications, and I know if and how they affect my sleep.

—— I take prescription medications or over-the-counter medications specifically to help me sleep.

—— I seem to have (or have been diagnosed with) a specific sleeping disorder, as described in chapter 3.

—— I have a medical condition that makes it difficult to sleep.

—— I know several things that I can do when I have trouble sleeping, and I feel that it's possible for them to work.

—— I am willing to do whatever it takes to improve my sleep.

Step Two: Make a Plan

Each one of these statements bears on some key area that affects sleep. According to your response, you can get a clear idea of what it is that may be causing the problem. Let's take each one in order and see if it's contributing to your sleepless nights. If it is, then there is always something you can do to change things.

I have made all the needed adjustments in my sleeping environment that can help me sleep better.

If you answered "no" to this statement, then this is where you begin if you want to improve the quality of your sleep. In the sleep potential inventory, several areas were mentioned that contribute to a poor sleeping environment. They included things like noise, bad mattresses, interruptions (like kids and pets) during the night, too much light, and more. The bald truth is this: if you don't fix these things, one way or another, you will not get the sleep you need. Solutions range from the simple to the complex, from earplugs to moving away. It's up to you to do it. Make a list of the things that don't work in your sleeping environment and then change them.

Some changes, like a new mattress, cost money. If money isn't readily available, make a plan to save the money you need—perhaps a small amount each week until you've accumulated enough. You will be so pleased by the results of sleeping on your new bed (or sleeping more peacefully as the result of some other expensive change, like installing an air conditioner) that you will quickly forget the struggle involved in getting the funds together.

You can do it, and you have only yourself to blame if you don't take the trouble required to make your sleeping environment as pleasant as possible. The benefits of improved sleep are great—better sleep, better health, and a better disposition as well.

If you responded with a "yes" to this statement, then good for you. This isn't the cause of the problem, and we can look elsewhere.

I understand the relationship of alcohol, nicotine, and caffeine to the quality of my sleep.

I hope you were able to say "yes" to this statement. What all of these substances have in common, of course, is the capacity to disturb or destroy sleep. You can't expect to have a drink, a cup of coffee, or a cigarette before going to bed and then get a restful night's sleep.

When I was a lot younger I used to do all of those things. I didn't think anything of it. I had that last cigarette and enjoyed it, got bombed once in a while and fell into bed, and I loved that cappuccino or espresso late at night. I wasn't smart enough or aware enough to realize how lousy my sleep was—I was just tired a lot or irritable, or not up to par with my work. I'd have another cigarette and attempt to relax. I was blessed with a strong body, so I blew off the many symptoms caused by poor sleeping habits.

Now I know better, and so does my body. If you are doing these things, try to alter your habits. Otherwise, you have to learn to do without good sleep, and that will affect everything else that you do. It will affect your judgment, your ability to think clearly, and your health, although you may not realize the real reason you keep getting all those colds and odd little illnesses. Loss of sleep has a direct impact on your immune system, leaving you more vulnerable to whatever comes along. You will not be at your best without enough sleep. If you don't care about being at your best, it's not an issue for you; don't worry about it. If it is, make the changes.

Probably the hardest of these sleep-destroying habits to shift is nicotine addiction, unless you are an alcoholic. Alcohol can be a nightmare, in every sense of the word. I'm not a preacher, and I'm not going to give a sermon about the evils of nicotine and alcohol. I've been there; I know what it's like. All I can say is that your sleep and your health demand that you give it up, one way or another.

If you have a problem with alcohol, bite the bullet and seek help. Alcoholics Anonymous works—so does private treatment. You are not alone, and you can find the courage to do it. If you're still a smoker, there are many programs to help you quit. Use them. No one can make you do it, but you will not believe the difference once you succeed in getting rid of the habit.

Make it your intention to change the habit that is ruining your sleep. If you need to stop smoking, talk with friends who have done it, or talk with your doctor. There are now several products on the market that can help you get rid of the physical addiction to nicotine, leaving only the psychological side of addiction to deal with.

If you are used to having a drink or two before bed, you are possibly at risk of alcoholism or alcohol addiction. Do you have other drinks earlier? How many? Do you drink every night before bed or only on occasion?

There's nothing wrong with an occasional drink, unless you happen to be allergic to alcohol. But if you take a look at your drinking habits and see that you are having several drinks, every day, you might pause and reflect. Sometimes you can head off a real problem by seeing the danger and cutting back. Sometimes the addiction is already there and must be dealt with through abstinence and treatment. If you think you have a problem, talk with your doctor or another counselor and seek advice about how to deal with it.

I understand the relationship of my eating habits and food preferences to the quality of my sleep.

You may have wondered exactly what I was getting at with this statement, since there is obviously such a diversity of thought and preference about food. Every culture is different, every individual is different, and everyone's tastes are different. If you answered "yes," then you can choose what and when to eat in a way that will not interfere with your sleep. You can choose to eat whatever you like before bed if you want to—as long as you understand the consequences of that late-night pizza.

If you responded with a "no," then you need to keep a simple fact in mind: overloading on food of any kind before bed is a sure recipe for sleeplessness and sleep disturbance. Some foods, like dairy products or potatoes, can actually help you sleep. But eating big helpings won't work. Late snacks have to be avoided, unless you are getting so hungry that it interferes with sleep. In that case, use common sense and avoid the spicy, acid, sugar-laden, or syrupy concoctions that may find their way to your bedside table.

Eating to sleep better is easy—it just requires a little common sense. If you have dinner at five in the evening and don't go to bed until eleven, you might get hungry before it's time to lie down. Have a snack around nine or nine-thirty, but don't load up on the chips or whatever after that. In fact, don't load up at all, and don't get suckered by those television ads that tell you can take a pill and avoid any problems with your digestion. (You know the ones I mean. Someone is gorging themselves on piles of hot and spicy foods, unconcerned about the havoc these foods can wreak. After all, they took the pill. If you do that, you are asking for trouble.)

Sleeping is not the right time for digesting. Remember that and don't create a sleep problem by asking your body to digest much while it's lying down.

I understand how circadian rhythms affect my sleep.

This statement is a little unfair, because there are still lots of unanswered questions about circadian rhythms. If you answered "no," you are in very good company. You don't have to be a sleep researcher, though, to have a sense of how the natural rhythms of daylight and darkness affect sleep. If you answered "yes," it probably means that you have a good understanding of how shift work, jet lag, and other disruptions in the normal day/night rhythm affects sleep.

You will recall that we talked about circadian rhythms in chapter 1, and that they are fundamental to our patterns of sleeping and waking. If you understand this, you can make any adjustments that might be necessary to help you through sleep problems caused by altering those rhythms. Like everything else, it requires your conscious attention and desire to make something happen.

If you know you're going to Tokyo or Hong Kong next week, prepare for the journey. Go to the extra effort it takes to adjust your cycle a little before you get there. Of course, if you are just going and flying right back, this might not be worth the trouble, unless it's absolutely essential that you be in top form for your meetings when you arrive. I know several people who travel frequently to distant countries. They are always talking about the effects and how tired they are. They also seem to find it impossible to make any preflight adjustment in their schedules. Their philosophy is to tough it out. I sympathize, but my sympathy is somewhat muted by knowing that they could make it easier on themselves if they really wanted to. It's your choice. Refer to chapter 1 for jet-lag advice.

Rotating shift changes are harder to deal with. See if you can at least set it up so that you are advancing in a clockwise direction as you rotate, *i.e.*, from night to early morning to afternoon. Try your best to get eight hours of sleep each day, no matter when you get off work. You may also want to think about getting a different job. I'm serious. What's it worth to you to have normal hours and normal sleep? Perhaps a better question is what are the consequences to you if you don't have enough sleep? For "normal sleep," read "good health."

The best strategy for dealing with circadian rhythms is to realize that they are a fundamental truth of our physical being, and that they cannot be ignored without consequences. Do the best you can, and realize that they must be honored, one way or another.

I think it's important to make enough time in my day to get a full eight hours of sleep.

If you said "yes," move on. If you said "no," I haven't made my point clear enough that eight hours is needed by most people. You might be one of the two percent or so that can get by on five and a half or six hours a night. If so, God bless you and skip ahead. But for almost all of the rest of us, six hours isn't going to cut it.

The problem, of course, is that we tend to get caught up in all of the many activities of work and play that fill up our lives. Our culture promotes this—countless variations of the "work hard, play hard" philosophy fill our work environments and our leisure time as well. Once we get hooked into this kind of lifestyle, time disappears. Work is especially to blame, since today's business environment seems to demand more and more of our time just to keep up and keep our jobs. We can't be blamed for wanting to spend some time having fun after the grind of daily work. Something has to give, and what usually goes by the board is sleep.

Once again, the only person who can change this is you. If you answered "no," it means that you just don't buy the need for adequate sleep and think you are the exception. I have unwelcome news for you: there are no exceptions. You can train yourself, within limits, to get by on less sleep, but that's just it—you are getting by, not getting sleep. Your sleep debt will accumulate and sneak up on you when you least expect it. Let's hope you will not be flying an airplane, driving a big semi on the interstate, or operating on me or someone I love when it does.

Take a look at your patterns of sleep and wakefulness. If you are consistently getting less than eight hours, you are most likely sleep deprived. Try to alter the pattern. If you are going to hang out on Friday and Saturday nights, don't plan a big event early on Sunday morning. Sleep in; try to catch up. Go to bed earlier on Sunday night. Try to keep on an even keel during the week and avoid the temptations that keep you up late, whatever they may be.

I know, I know, it's not always easy. I'm not trying to be a complete party-pooper here. Just do the best you can, and make an effort to program eight hours into your busy schedule for the rest and sleep you need. You'll be glad you did.

I make sure that I take time to relax and let go of daily problems and worries.

A "no" answer means you are probably somewhat stressed and probably caught up in too many things to do without enough time to do them. This kind of constant stress is very common; it is also a widespread cause of sleeplessness. If this is true for you, take a look at all of those activities. Something can surely be eliminated, freeing up some time to just let it all go and relax. Even if you are very busy, making time to relax is a choice you can make.

We are always making choices, often without being fully aware of why we are making them. Even hard-headed business managers have come to recognize the need for regular down time on a daily basis, time to let go of some of the stress and do nothing but relax. Most time management courses will include a talk about handling stress and scheduling time to relax during the day. Make a choice to take time to relax, either during the day or sometime in the evening.

Here's a simple exercise to help clear your mind during the day or before bed. You can do this about a half-hour or so before bedtime, or anytime that you can make fifteen minutes or so available. Experiment until you get the right timing for you.

Into the Pool

—— Get comfortable in a quiet place, such as your bedroom, your office (this will work during the day to reduce stress—not for sleep but for relaxation) or wherever you can be comfortable. It is critical that you be sure you won't be disturbed.

—— Close your eyes and take a few deep breaths. It helps to inhale deeply through your nose and exhale through your mouth. Let the air escape with a soft whooshing sound.

—— Imagine, in your mind's eye, that you are seated on the banks of a beautiful pool, one with clear, deep water. The water flows away from you and out of the end of the pool, over a pleasant waterfall. Imagine the feel of the air, the sound of the water, the clearness of the day. Feel the sun on your face, smell the grass, the

188

trees, and the flowers. Make the image as real as possible. Take your time.

——— Now let your thoughts about all the things you have to do come up in your mind. Just give them a minute or so to get going. Notice that there always seems to be lots of things to do.

——— Make an agreement with yourself. In your mind, tell yourself that you will get to these things and that you will make sure that they get done. If your mind insists on going into detail, politely and firmly tell yourself that you will get it done, and you can be trusted to do it. (I know this sounds silly, but our minds are like this—it's as if we were several people at once, arguing over the best way to do something.)

——— Now pick a thought about something you have to do, and imagine that it is like a piece of colored paper. The thing that needs to be done is like a piece of colored paper. Take the piece of paper and crumple it up into a ball, and toss it into the pool. Notice how the gentle current in the pool catches the paper and moves it toward the waterfall. Watch the paper drift with the current across the pool, until it disappears over the edge of the falls.

——— Do the same thing with each thought about something that needs to be done. Imagine that it is a piece of colored paper, crumple it up into a ball, toss it into the pool, and watch it drift away over the edge of the falls.

——— When you have gone through all of the things that need to be done, imagine yourself sitting quietly for a few moments by the edge of the water. Then take a few deep breaths and open your eyes.

This visualization exercise takes a little practice. Go easy and let it take a natural shape in your mind's eye. The setting can be anywhere, and you may find that you are imagining something different from what I have described here. That's okay. Take the image you get and let the things you have to do gently disappear. At the end of the day, this exercise can help you calm your mind for sleep.

I take prescription medications, and I know if and how they affect my sleep.

There isn't any way that I can adequately cover the possibilities of prescription medications affecting your sleep in this book. If you have trouble sleeping and are taking prescription drugs, you need to be able to respond with "yes" to this statement. If not, perhaps the meds are contributing to the sleep problem. You need to find out, so ask your doctor or pharmacist. You can also look up your medications in the *Physician's Desk Reference* and find out if there are possible side effects affecting your sleep. This book can be found in your local library or a large bookstore. Make sure it's up to date. If you have any questions, it's back to your doctor or pharmacist again. They have to keep up with the latest drugs, especially at the pharmacy.

Make a list of what you are taking and go get the information you need. Some common drugs, like inhalants for asthma or drugs for high blood pressure can affect sleep. You can often counteract negative sleep effects by making sure that everything else in your sleep situation is as ideal as possible and by following the general guidelines, like avoiding alcohol and caffeine. If the problem continues, talk with your doctor.

I take prescription or over-the-counter medications specifically to help me sleep.

Chapter 5 contains a lot of information about OTC and prescription sleeping drugs. If you responded with "yes" to this question, please pay close attention to what has been said there. All sleeping drugs are potentially dangerous to your health or disruptive to your normal and healthy sleep. They can be a wonderful temporary fix to break a cycle of sleeplessness; they can easily become a curse. Avoid them if possible, and consider some of the herbal alternatives.

If you are taking these drugs, make a plan to get off them. Talk with your doctor if you are taking prescription sleeping aids. Use the information in this book to discover why you are not sleeping in the first place and to correct whatever is needed to bring back normal sleep.

I seem to have (or have been diagnosed with) a specific sleeping disorder, as described in chapter 3.

If you think that you have a sleeping disorder (like apnea or restless leg syndrome), see your doctor. If you have already been diagnosed with a sleep disorder, learn everything you can about it, and do what is needed to correct it. Your doctor can put you in touch with a specialist who works with sleep problems or refer you to a sleep disorder center near you. Aside from the large, research-oriented facilities like Stanford University, UCLA, or the University of Chicago, many major hospitals now have some kind of sleep-disorder program. A brief list of some major sleep-disorder centers and other sleep resources is given at the end of this book.

A sleep disorder is like any other health problem. It must be treated, and it needs professional and competent oversight by someone who is trained in the best ways to deal with the problem. You can't usually fix one of these by yourself. Some of them are life threatening, so take steps to address the issue.

I have a medical condition that makes it difficult to sleep.

This is a tough one. There is no simple fix to handle sleep problems caused by things like severe chronic pain, serious illnesses like cancer, or some other medical problem that wrecks sleep. I hope you were able to say "no" to this one and move on. If not, I have a couple of suggestions.

General, overall comfort is critical, no matter what the problem. That means clean, smooth sheets, the right kinds of foods and nutrition, and a peaceful environment. It means massage, if needed, and lotions to soothe tired and dry skin. It means making an effort to take charge of your environment in a way that supports more comfort and better sleep. That can be a real problem for someone who is seriously ill.

Chronic pain has to be addressed, one way or another. Biofeedback techniques can be very effective and are completely natural, requiring no drugs. Remember that our brain waves change when we start the process of going to sleep. The busy and fast beta waves change to alpha waves, which are slower and of longer duration. With biofeedback, the patient learns to adjust his or her internal rhythms. Typically, blood pressure is lowered, stress levels drop dramatically, and a pattern of alpha waves appears, resulting in a calm state of mind and a reduction in perceived pain.

One common biofeedback device measures levels of galvanic skin response (GSR) and uses this to trigger a continuous sound. The changing pitch of the sound lets the operator know whether or not he or she is succeeding in calming things down. GSR can be considered as a measure of stress. For example, variations in GSR are recorded during a lie detector test, indicating stress levels in the subject and, presumably, lies or the lack of them. By learning how to consciously calm the body and mind and reduce the amount of "charge" in the GSR, patients can learn to modify and even eliminate their sensations of pain. They can alter their experience. Biofeedback practitioners and technicians are trained in a variety of techniques they can use to help clients achieve control over things like high blood pressure and chronic pain.

I like biofeedback because it is self-empowering, always available, and under personal control. This may be a good option for you to explore. There are books on the subject available either at the library or at your local bookstore, if you would like to learn more.

I think there is an excellent option for supporting people who have chronic pain or serious illness, but it is not always understood or supported by all caregivers. That option is hypnotherapy. A competent and well-trained hypnotherapist can help you learn to control and moderate pain. A good hypnotherapist may also be able to alleviate pain on the spot. Hypnotherapy can be used to moderate and reduce the side effects of treatments like chemotherapy or dialysis.

Hypnotherapy is a growing profession, and there is a wide spectrum of credibility and competence among practitioners. Training ranges from minimal to extensive. Look for a hypnotherapist who has at least been certified by a national organization, such as the National Guild of Hypnotists. Look for other credentials of education and training as well. A personal recommendation from a friend who has worked with someone is good, if you can get one. Your doctor may know of someone.

As always, you must feel comfortable with the person you choose. Ask as many questions as you need to, and expect clear answers. Most therapists will offer an initial appointment at no cost, in order to see if there is a good fit between client and practitioner and to answer questions, schedule appointments, and establish fees. It usually is best to think in terms of several sessions, not just one. It takes time to build rapport and establish trust. If you decide to try hypnosis, give it a fair try and don't expect miracles the first time you talk with someone.

The self-hypnosis technique given in chapter 7 can be modified to help you support yourself in receiving treatment or feeling more comfortable in your body. Try it. You have nothing to lose.

I know several things that I can do when I have trouble sleeping, and I feel that it's possible for them to work.

This one has to be met with a "yes" if you have really paid attention while reading this book. I don't think you would have gotten this far if you weren't convinced that it's possible to affect your sleep and didn't want to learn what to do and how to do it. If you said "no," it's possible you are just a little depressed about the whole thing and don't find it easy to be optimistic. That is a typical sign of sleep deprivation, so perhaps you are simply responding out of that sense of inner exhaustion that comes from poor sleep and mounting sleep debt.

There are many things you can do when you have trouble sleeping; this book is full of them. Make a list, and then do whatever seems to be required. It's a bit like the "just do it" Nike philosophy, but sometimes that really is the best approach. You can do it.

I am willing to do whatever it takes to improve my sleep.

This last statement is in some ways the most important. In the end, there is only one person who can help you to sleep more soundly and to get the rest you deserve. That person is you. You may need advice, you may need a prescription, and you may need to make changes in your life and in your living or sleeping environment. Whatever it is, you are the only one who can make it happen.

If you are not willing to do what it takes, why are you reading this book?

SLEEP WELL, SLEEP DEEP

I'd like to end this book with a vision for you to consider, a dream that can become real. In this dream you don't experience any problem sleeping. In fact, in this dream you sleep so well and so deeply that it almost amazes you when people tell you how tired they are or how they have been spending so many sleepless nights. You can sympathize with their plight, but for you it's different. When you get ready for bed, it's in anticipation of a peaceful, relaxing night. You fall asleep almost as soon as your head touches the pillow. You sleep through the night. Perhaps you wake briefly once or twice, but it's not a problem: you quickly and easily fall back asleep. When you awaken in the morning you feel refreshed and alert, ready to begin your day and meet the wonderful possibilities that life offers.

Sound like a dream? It can become your reality, if you set your desire and intention to make it so. Your natural state of being includes sound and peaceful sleep. In our modern society things are far from being in a natural state. We have to adapt and learn to make our own island of calm sanity in the midst of the chaos around us. Deep sleep is the key to many other things: better health, happiness and well-being, better relationships, improved abilities, and a cheerful disposition are all founded on deep sleep. Sleep alone will not make us happy, but without sleep, happiness will almost surely elude our outstretched hand.

Please use the ideas and information in this book to add to your enjoyment of life and to your personal sense of well-being. May you sleep well, sleep deep.

ACKNOWLEDGMENTS

When you stop and think about it, the nature of sleep research often makes it impossible to get a good night's sleep or maintain a decent schedule of study, work, rest, and relaxation. When everyone else is happily asleep, the unheralded researcher is keeping an eye on things and hoping something—anything—might happen to interrupt the monotony. It seems to me that watching people sleep is a lot like watching paint dry. It's not very exciting, and it takes a lot of dedication.

It would not be possible to write a book like this without referring to the work of others. The bibliography in the back reflects that reality, but I thought I'd mention a few people here. Their work has become an integrated part of the body of human knowledge and is the foundation of any attempt to understand the nature and mechanisms of sleep. Even though *Sleep Well, Sleep Deep* is not a "technical" book in the academic sense, the work of these folks has influenced and shaped some of the content.

Dr. Nathaniel Klietman of the University of Chicago was the first to make sleep a respectable and valuable field of serious scientific study. Dr. William Dement of Stanford University, another true pioneer, is a good candidate for the title of Guru of American Sleep Studies. Dr. Peretz Lavie, of the Technion Institute in Israel, deserves special mention. Dr. Ernest Hartmann, of Yale University, has contributed much to academic sleep literature. Dr. Stanley Coren, of British Columbia, helped bring the mystery of sleep into the public eye with his book *The Sleep Thieves*.

In addition to the work of these men, I also freely used the Internet in my research. A few, key, non-commercial and medical site addresses are given in the back of the book. There is a lot of information to be found by reading through some of the commercial sites, particularly when it comes to supplements that can aid sleep, like L-tryptophan. As I do not wish to promote any products, I have not listed them. They cover the whole gamut from very small firms to large drug manufacturers. It is necessary to take the information provided by the commercial sites with several grains of salt. Nonetheless, these sites can provide valuable information. Just remember that they would like to sell you something. You can find them with your Internet search engine.

Special mention to my wife, Gayle, and to Noah, Mark, Bill, John, Wewer, and Brugh.

Thank you.

RESOURCES

The American Sleep Disorders Association is an association of doctors and professionals who specialize in sleep medicine and sleep disorders. If you have Internet access, the Web site address for the ASDA is: http://www.asda.org. The site has a very complete list of centers throughout the country. Currently, every state except Wyoming has at least one accredited sleep-disorder center. The ASDA provides free information and helpful pamphlets upon request. You can write to them at

> American Sleep Disorders Association
> 6301 Bandel Road, Suite 101
> Rochester, MN 55901

Major hospitals, especially in large urban areas, often have a sleep-disorder program. Some universities with medical schools have sleep labs and programs for treating sleep disorders. You can also find private sleep-disorder centers listed on the Internet. Use your search engine, and you will be rewarded with many choices and a ton of information.

For information on finding a sleep-disorder center near you, you can also write to

> Association of Sleep Disorder Centers
> c/o Sleep Disorder Clinic
> Stanford University School of Medicine
> Stanford, CA 94305

Sleep Well, Sleep Deep

The National Sleep Foundation is a good place to start for any questions or information about sleep and sleeping disorders. You can contact the foundation at

National Sleep Foundation
1522 K Street NW
Suite 510
Washington, DC 20005

202-347-3471

Their Web address is http://www.sleepfoundation.org and their e-mail address is natsleep@arrows.com. Their website has a wonderful series of links that can take you to more specific areas of interest, including links to Germany and Canada and to organizations like the Narcolepsy Network or the American Sleep Apnea Association.

BIBLIOGRAPHY

Carskadon, M. A. *Encyclopedia of Sleep and Dreaming*. New York: Macmillan, 1993.

Coren, S. *The Sleep Thieves*. New York: The Free Press, 1996.

Dement, W. C. *The Sleepwatchers*. Stanford, Calif.: Stanford Alumni Association, 1992.

Ford, N. *Good Night*. Gloucester, Mass.: Para Research, Inc., 1983.

Hartmann, E. L. *The Functions of Sleep*. New Haven and London: Yale University Press, 1973.

Hollyer, B., and Smith, L. *The Secret of Problem-Free Nights*. London: Ward Lock, 1996.

Klietman, N. *Sleep and Wakefulness*. Chicago: University of Chicago Press, 1963.

Lavie, P. *The Enchanted World of Sleep*. New Haven: Yale University Press, 1996.

INTERNET REFERENCES

*T*here are many, many sites on the Internet containing information on everything concerning sleep. The Net has become a primary research tool, and I used it freely during the writing of this book. For example, some of the information on herbs and on the composition and effects of some prescription drugs was obtained on the Net. The information gathered added to what I already knew or expanded my knowledge in some way. I am going to list a few major sites here that provided information I found useful and informative. The information they contained contributed to the writing of this book, just as the conventional sources of written material did, and I want to acknowledge that fact. Perhaps you will find them helpful as well.

The Mayo Clinic. Good for information on an enormous number of health problems, including sleep disorders and complications arising from poor sleep.

http://www.mayohealth.org

Botanical.com. Very complete on-line herbal encyclopedia, with just about everything you need to know about different herbs. Not a commercial site, just a labor of love by a lady named Mrs. M. Grieve. Highly recommended if you are interested in herbs.

http://www.botanical.com

Article by Dr. P.J. Cowen. Excellent article by Dr. Cowen about serotonin and depression. Although the focus is on depression, the information about tryptophan, serotonin, etc., is up to date and useful.

http://www.depression.org.uk

California State University, Chico. The university has a series of Web pages under the heading of Biological Psychology. Good for information about neurotransmitters.

http://www.csuchico.edu/psy/BioPsych

National Institutes of Health Consensus Development Conference. An article entitled *Drugs and Insomnia: The Use of Medications to Promote Sleep*. Technical and informative.

http://text.nlm.nih.gov/nih/cdc/www/39txt.html

Colorado Health Net. An article entitled *Overview of Foods and Drugs That May Promote Sleep*. This is primarily directed at health care professionals who are working with cancer patients. Very informative. If you or someone you know suffers from cancer, check this one out.

http://www.coloradohealthnet.org/sleep/sleep_ncimed.html

INDEX

ABS. *See* automatic behavior syndrome
acid reflux, 137
acupressure, 119
acupuncture, 83, 87, 119, 134, 136
addiction, 50, 66, 114, 128, 183, 184
adenoids, 160
adolescents, 107, 162, 163
alcohol, 9, 19, 22, 31-32, 46, 50, 54, 59, 69, 76, 79, 86, 100, 116-117, 123, 137, 180, 182-184, 190
alcoholism, 55, 87, 183-184
Alexander Technique, 134
all-heal. *See* valerian
alpha waves, 11-13, 192
amino acids, 10, 28, 119, 123
American Massage and Therapy Association, 133
anesthesiology, 17, 20
animals, 12-13, 41, 100, 167
antihistamines, 19, 117
apartments, 8, 53-54, 67
apnea, 60-61, 73, 83-86, 116, 138, 147, 160, 191
aspirin, 40, 46
asthma, 51, 100, 113, 118, 190
Atkins, Robert C., 132
auto-suggestion, 175

automatic behavior syndrome, 17
Ayurvedic medicine, 43

babies, 141-150, 157-158
barbiturates, 114
bed-wetting, 158
bedtime rituals, 70-71, 75, 145
beer, 21, 131, *see also* alcohol
benzodiazepines, 114, 115, 116, 130
beta waves, 11-13, 192
biofeedback, 12, 79, 192
biological clock, 13, 26, 28, 163
bladder, 51, 59, 158
Braid, James, 167, 168
brain lesions, 82
brain waves, 11, 12, 168, 192
breathing, 18, 34, 35, 36, 37, 43, 44, 60, 61, 74, 83, 84, 85, 101, 113, 118, 170, 171, 173, 174, 188

caffeine, 19, 33, 51, 65, 137, 180, 182, 190
calcium, 138
calm, 12, 33-34, 37, 40-41, 43-44, 49, 66, 70-71, 75, 77, 90, 119, 122, 128, 130-131, 141, 146, 153, 154, 158, 170, 176, 190, 192, 195

Index

Index